The Non-Stop Paleo Life

The Non-Stop Paleo Life

HOW TO HACK YOUR WAY TO A HEALTHIER LIFE

Dr. Nick Caras

Dedication and Acknowledgment

To my beautiful wife: Thank you for allowing us to raise our family through a different health-care lens than most. Living a Paleo way of life is not always the easiest as it takes planning, willpower, and doing what's best for our children, but you always seem to make it happen.

To Alex and P: This book is for you. I hope that someday you will carry forward the same passion as I have for the health-and-wellness lifestyle that you are growing up in.

Table of Contents

Preface: The Paleo Chiropractor

The marriage between the Paleo lifestyle and the chiropractic lifestyle is a match made in heaven. When I was in chiropractic college in the early 2000s, chiropractic philosophy was a brand-new paradigm for me. Like many, I entered chiropractic college after finishing my premed degree because I wanted to help people with back injuries and different sorts of sports injuries. I soon found out that chiropractic was never really meant to treat back injuries, sciatica, herniated discs, headaches, migraines, and back pain.

Little did I know I was in for that rude awakening. Chiropractic was founded in 1895 because the first chiropractic adjustment, performed by D. D. Palmer, actually restored a deaf man's hearing back to normal. Dr. Palmer knew that there was a link between the brain and spinal cord and all the different functions of the body. If we could take pressure off this pathway (now known as your nervous system), we could help the body heal and restore normal function. In the earliest case, doing so helped a deaf man start to hear again.

I quickly learned in my early years of graduate school that this brain/body link was a huge part of being healthy. Chiropractic college also taught me that health comes from within us and not from outside sources like medication, surgery, or radiation. There has not been and never will be a magic pill that will restore health to a diseased body.

Throughout my years of chiropractic college and other postgraduate degrees in wellness and nutrition, I was drawn to the teachings of Dr. Loren Cordain of Colorado State University. He had been studying the people of the Paleolithic Era and noticed how healthy they were. They were mostly free of cancer, heart disease, cavities, clogged arteries, obesity, arthritis, and other lifestyle diseases that plague America today. He was really onto something. He wanted to find out how these people were living and what they were doing differently from modern humankind. He asked himself, *What is the key to living a life free of all these diseases?* The answer became the Paleo diet as we know it today.

As it turns out, the modern Paleo lifestyle is very similar to the lifestyle that chiropractors have been teaching since the early 1900s.

The goal of this book is to teach you my version of this lifestyle and what it looks like in today's fast-paced era. As the title shows, I call this lifestyle the *"Non-Stop Paleo Lifestyle."* You see, I am a husband, a father of two beautiful girls, a full-time chiropractic physician, a health coach, and an author. My point is, I am busy just like you! Yet my family and I live a very healthy lifestyle without breaking the bank. There is no need to drive through your local fast-food burger joint for dinner just because you are busy. With a little commitment and planning, you too can live the Non-Stop Paleo Lifestyle.

The reason I chose the name *"Non-Stop Paleo"* is that I want this lifestyle to be yours for the rest of your life. My lifestyle has built-in cheat days and reward days, so you can splurge a little bit. After all, you only live once, and I truly believe that we should be able to have a few cheat days here and there. Throughout my years in private practice and having consulted with thousands of patients from around the world, I have come to the conclusion that if you take away everything a patient loves 100 percent of the time, the patient will never stick with the program. Again, this is **non-stop**: it is meant to be a lifestyle and not another fad diet or quick weight-loss program.

Every choice you make is either moving you closer to health or closer to disease.
—Dr. Nick Caras

I truly hope you enjoy this program as I know it will make a huge difference in your overall health, happiness, and longevity. Also, please make this a family affair. There is nothing more gratifying to me as a physician than seeing an entire family live a healthy and happy lifestyle.

This book is just the beginning. It is meant to get you and your loved ones off on the right foot. This book is not the be-all and end-all. There will be a lot of work ahead of you. Once you get the major premise down and start living the Paleo way, you will want so much more.

As you read through this book, check out my accompanying website at **www.NonStopPaleo.com** for recipes, paleohacks, motivation, research, and everything Paleo. This is a journey; it starts with getting the concepts I am about to lay out for you with this book, and the end game is to continue to read and self-motivate about the Paleo lifestyle.

In my experience, once my patients and private clients adopt this lifestyle, they absolutely love the results and fall in love with learning more. You may find it a little unfamiliar in the beginning, and the lifestyle planning and preparation may catch you off guard, but like anything new, if you just stick with it for a couple weeks, it all becomes habit. Results will speak for themselves and keep you on track. There is nothing better than losing weight, having more energy, feeling better, and being happier to keep you on track and motivated!

CHAPTER 1

The Non-Stop Paleo Life Premise

Science and research are always expanding in the health-care arena, and we're always gaining new insights and new scientific literature. This "new" concept of Non-Stop Paleo has been an ongoing lifestyle for me, and later my entire family, for over fifteen years.

In the Paleo world, we sometimes call our practice *biohacking*. For example, if new research comes out on a certain supplement, a certain food group, or a new way to exercise or sleep, we'll self-experiment (biohack) and see what changes, good or bad, come of it. We may notice better cellular function, increased weight loss, fewer digestive issues, better blood work results, and so forth.

Over many years of reading about new scientific research in medical journals; postgraduate courses in nutrition, wellness, and brain function; and biohacking, I started to compile lists of what moves someone toward health or away from health (toward disease)—no matter how old or young you are.

Certain ways of exercising will make you healthy, and other ways actually cause diseases such as arthritis, heart disease, and immune deficiencies and will age you much more quickly than normal.

The goal and mission of this book as well as the Non-Stop Paleo Lifestyle are to show you exactly what will move you and your family toward healthy childhood development, continued good health, longevity, and graceful aging as well as move you away from chronic diseases and increased rates of aging. The most significant keyword and takeaway I want for you is "non-stop"; this is truly a program for the rest of your life. No matter how old you are right now, you can start this lifestyle. The Non-Stop Paleo Life is also meant to be easy to implement, affordable, and a usable method for your entire family.

If you're in your sixties and near retirement, you can start the Non-Stop Paleo Lifestyle and reap the benefits well into your retirement years. If you're in your thirties or forties, this book can be life-changing, as you have a large portion of your working life still in front of you. Implement the strategies right now, and you'll see all sorts of benefits, from weight loss and increased work productivity to being a better spouse and parent to increased energy and better sleep.

If you're a parent, you can change your kids' lives profoundly. Teach them now how to live a healthier and more active lifestyle, and they'll be set up to succeed in every aspect of life from school to sports, their work ethic, and their respect levels.

90/10 Rule: Putting the "Non-Stop" in Non-Stop Paleo

With the non-stop aspect of this lifestyle comes a rule I want you to live by: the 90/10 rule. Many of you are probably familiar with the more common 80/20 rule in different aspects of your lives. It's when you do something good 80 percent of the time and maybe cheat a little bit 20 percent of the time. In business, we sometimes use the 80/20 rule to do our most productive strategies 80 percent of the time and then some fun strategies that may not be as productive in our business lives 20 percent of the time.

Some of you may use the 80/20 rule for your home finances or budgeting. For example, when you find yourself with discretionary income or some leftover money at the end of the month, you may put

80 percent into a savings plan and then splurge on a new toy or a nice dinner with the remaining 20 percent. You get the idea.

With the Non-Stop Paleo Lifestyle, I want to up the ante a little bit. I would like you to live by the health strategies that I lay out in this book 90 percent of the time and then allow yourself to cheat or splurge 10 percent of the time. Does that sound fair enough to you? You'll end up being extremely healthy, but at the same time, you'll get to enjoy life along with some splurges and cheat meals throughout the week.

In my thirteen years of private practice and helping thousands of patients from around the world, I've met few who walk the walk and talk the talk 100 percent of the time. Most are lying if they tell you they never cheat, never take a day off from the gym, and are always super positive and in the right mind-set.

Again, I want this new lifestyle to be easily sustainable for you and your family. This isn't another fad diet or weight-loss program; this is where true health and well-being come from.

> *The secret of getting ahead is simply*
> *getting started.*
> *—Mark Twain*

So that's the key: the 90/10 rule. It's up to you how you want to play with it. Simply put, a lot of my patients and clients throughout the years have made a Saturday or Sunday a cheat day. Others, like many of my busy business professionals, make it a weekday-evening cheat meal because they're consistently at different work functions or traveling for business throughout the week. I'll also show you how to travel, fly, and stay at hotels while maintaining the Non-Stop Paleo Life on the run.

The strategies are so simple that you can implement them as part of virtually any routine, schedule, family, or work environment and all the lifestyles you may live within. There really won't be any more excuses for not being healthy and illness-free.

If you're sick and tired of feeling sick and tired day in and day out, then it's definitely time to change. Read through this book and start to implement the strategies today. No more excuses and no more yo-yo dieting. The new you starts today!

Action Steps
Respond to the following:

Why do you want to be healthy?

_____

_____

_____

Write down your number-one motivating factor.

_____

_____

_____

Do you want to be healthy for you or for someone else?

_____

_____

Purchase a journal and each morning write out the main reasons why you want to live a healthier life and one habit you plan on implementing that day. For example, "I will drink a minimum of 8 glasses of water today."

CHAPTER 2

Dietary Inflammation and What It Means for Your Body

et's face it: most of the modern world's chronic/lifestyle diseases are caused by the underlying problem known as *inflammation*. We've all heard this word before, but what does it really mean? If you've ever sprained your ankle or your knee, you know what acute inflammation is, but chronic inflammation is a whole different ball game.

Chronic inflammation is a low-grade, silent condition in which the body loses its ability to shut down. Not to be confused with a swollen ankle joint, where a little ice and rest does the trick and you're back to normal in no time, chronic inflammation is always present, constantly wearing down your cells, blood vessels, organs, and tissues and overall just aging you quicker than you should age. You really don't feel this chronic inflammation, but research now shows it's a big cause of all our American lifestyle diseases, such as heart disease, arthritis, cancer, diabetes, autoimmune diseases, obesity, high cholesterol, fatigue, and chronic pain.

The number-one reason why we need to adopt more of a Paleo way of life is that our Paleolithic ancestors didn't have all these chronic diseases. In fact, they were virtually free of the major American lifestyle diseases mentioned above.

How were these people who lived so long ago free of chronic back pain, heart disease, strokes, cancer, and the like? The answer is actually simple: they didn't have the constant levels of chronic inflammation that most of us have today in twenty-first century. To take it a step further, it's because they didn't eat and drink all the chemical-laden items that are in the standard American diet.

Simple concept, right? Well, not really. Even if we started to eat more fruits, vegetables, and other whole foods from our local grocery store and stopped eating packaged baked goods and sodas, there's still a problem:

Toxins are lurking in every corner of our kitchens and causing cellular inflammation every day inside our bodies.
—Dr. Nick Caras

More chemicals are on and, more importantly, inside our foods than at any other time in history. Whether crops are sprayed with pesticides, fungicides, or herbicides or are genetically modified, chemicals are getting inside you one way or another.

Research has shown that our obesity epidemic in America is actually a toxicity epidemic. We're filled with toxic chemicals from our infancy through childhood and into adulthood. We breathe them in, eat and drink them, rub them on our skin through lotions and antiperspirants, put them on our lawns, and even cook and store our food inside them. Medical studies have shown that most toxic chemicals can get into our brains and even pass through placenta into our babies.

We must start living a more organic, natural, and green lifestyle to reach our full health potential. A huge part of the Non-Stop Paleo Lifestyle is learning how to shop organic with regard to your food choices and cleaning products as well as how to perform daily, weekly, and yearly detoxes to ensure a clean body inside and out.

In my eight-week Non-Stop Paleo Lifestyle program, I go through each protocol for how to properly detox and continually flush out toxins. (To learn more about the Non-Stop Paleo Boot Camp eight-week program, check out www.nonstoppaleo.com/paleo-lifestyle-8-week-bootcamp/.

There's no getting around it. We live in such a toxic world that detoxification protocols aren't a luxury but a necessity. If you choose not to detoxify regularly, chronic inflammation will continue to mount inside your body until your body can't handle it anymore, at which time disease will soon follow.

Let's backtrack for a moment and talk about some of the most inflammatory foods. These are the foods that you should never (or rarely) consume.

Read that again: These are the foods you should never (or rarely) consume.

Inflammatory Foods

Gluten
Sugar
Alcohol
Dairy
Grains
Conventionally Raised Meat
Vegetable Oils
Processed Grains and Cereals
Wheat
Cookies, Cakes, and Other Desserts
Sugary drinks, including soda, sport drinks,
energy drinks, beer, wine, and liquors.
Breads, Processed Grains and Cereals, and **Wheat**,
including muffins, pancakes, waffles, baked goods,

> pizza crusts, pita breads, wheat chips, crackers, and
> pretzels; you get the point here—breads are bad.

All these foods and beverages are very inflammatory to your body. The most havoc and inflammation wrought by these foods actually take place inside your digestive tract. Your gut is home to billions of bacteria. Some are good, health-promoting bacteria (probiotic bacteria), and others are nasty, disease-causing bacteria. By eating these inflammatory foods, you will start to diminish the good probiotic bacteria, and this will leave room for the nasty, bad bacteria to thrive. When this imbalance happens, your body and your immune system will become weak and disease will start to set in. You will be more prone to colds, flus, cancers, and other lifestyle diseases.

It's time to eliminate these inflammatory foods in your diet. It is actually fairly simple to start to eliminate these inflammatory and processed foods. You just need to have the education and willpower to start living a more natural, whole-foods diet. The *Non-Stop Paleo Diet* gives you the tools you need to do this. Once you dive in, you will feel so energized and replenished that when you do have an inflammatory meal, you will really feel the effects it has on your body, and this will deter you from eating similar foods in the future.

Or perhaps you will find you can tolerate the 90 percent/10 percent way of life. For example, if you are out for pizza with your kid's flag football team, just make sure you eat a salad first, drink lots of water, enjoy one slice of pizza, and call it a night. This way you are hydrating the body and getting tons of good fiber, vegetables, and anti-inflammatory nutrients from the salad, and this allows your body to not be completely overwhelmed by "pizza night." Take it a step further: add a bunch of vegetables to your pizza and opt for thin crust (less bread) instead of going for the regular crust and a "meat-lovers" pie. Do you get the point here? You still have the capacity to enjoy life, but you'll be enjoying a healthier version of life. I love it when patients and clients tell me they didn't have to change much, but these little changes allowed them to lose weight (and keep it off), feel better, have more energy, and just have more self-esteem. These little tricks go such a long way in the lives of individuals and their families!

Those of you who are already familiar with the core principles of the Paleo diet know to stay away from dairy and grains. This is where this whole "Paleo thing" started; researchers became aware of how detrimental dairy foods and grain foods were to your body. If you just do these two steps, you will overcome many sicknesses and diseases, but if you follow the entire *Non-Stop Paleo Lifestyle*, you will be taking your health and longevity to a whole different level! I seriously urge you to eliminate these inflammatory food groups today and get on more of a whole-food, vegetable-based, clean-protein, and healthy-fat diet. This is the *Non-Stop Paleo Diet*!

Action Steps
Clean Out Your Kitchen: Throw Out Your Inflammatory Foods TODAY!

- Get rid of breads, pastas, rice, and cereals.
- Get rid of dairy products: milk and cheese.
- Eliminate alcohol or reduce intake to just one serving a week.
- Get rid of your inflammatory vegetable oils, and replace with healthy oils like olive oil and coconut oils.
- Eliminate conventionally raised meats, and only purchase grass-fed meats, poultry, and eggs.
- Start to consume water, tea, and black coffee exclusively—no other beverages.

Whether you think you can, or you think you cannot—you're probably right.
—Henry Ford

Most people like to procrastinate on throwing their inflammatory foods into the trash can. I challenge you to go into your cupboard and fridge right now and get this step done. It will make a huge difference in your life and shift your mentality to know these foods are no longer acceptable.

CHAPTER 3

Eating the Non-Stop Paleo Way

OK, guys, here we go! What are you going to eat day in and day out? This is one of my favorite topics to talk to patients about. No matter what condition, symptom, or disease you may be suffering from, we need to start to heal you by looking at what you are eating throughout your day.

> *Let Food Be Your Medicine, and Medicine
> Be Your Food.*
> *—Hippocrates, 400 BCE*

Anti-Inflammatory Foods

Kale
Spinach
Arugula
Broccoli
Asparagus
Blueberries
Tea

Cauliflower
Onions
Mushrooms
Garlic
Red and Orange Bell Peppers
Wild-Caught Salmon

Anti-Inflammatory Spices

Turmeric
Ginger
Cayenne
Cloves
Rosemary
Allspice
Oregano
Sage
Marjoram
Thyme

If I had to sum this up fairly quickly, I would tell you to eat a lot of vegetables throughout the day, a ton of healthy fat, a little bit of protein, and lots of clean water. This may not sound great at first glance, but trust me, the food options and meal-planning possibilities are endless. Once you really dive into the *Non-Stop Paleo* way of eating, your options become delicious and extremely healthy! You will never run out of food choices, recipes, and meal plans. Like most of us, you will have your seven to fifteen staple breakfasts, lunches, and dinners. Believe it or not, most of us eat the same thing week after week and month after month. With that in mind, this is not going to be too difficult to come up with your meals after I teach you the proper ingredients.

Breakfast
Staple Breakfast Ingredients

- Eggs from free-range chickens
- Avocados
- Mushrooms
- Bell peppers
- Tomatoes
- Spinach
- Onions
- Greek yogurt made from coconut or almond milk
- Organic bacon
- Grass-fed sausage links or patties (or chorizo)
- Sweet potatoes or yams
- Bulletproof Coffee (to be discussed later)
- Coconut oil
- Fresh berries
- Coconut milk
- Almond milk

Non-Stop Paleo Breakfast Meals

- Scrambled eggs with sautéed veggies and one breakfast meat from above
- Veggie omelets with sliced avocado
- Strawberry and blueberry parfait with coconut-milk yogurt
- Paleo quiche (a.k.a. crustless quiche) with mushrooms and peppers and a side of berries
- Baked sweet potato stuffed with scrambled eggs and bacon
- Hard-boiled eggs with sliced avocado and fresh berries
- Protein/fruit smoothie (water, frozen berries, spinach, avocado; options are endless for healthy breakfast smoothies.)

- Breakfast frittata with spinach, chives, and scallions
- Paleo Mexican omelet, including grape tomatoes, red onion, and chives, topped with avocado slices and cilantro

I hope you get the picture here. You can obviously mix and match these ingredients however you would like. A couple rules of thumb I would keep in mind are the following: First, to always use coconut oil in your pan or skillet when making scrambled eggs or omelets. Second, I would try to throw in some avocado every single morning, whether you would like to simply eat one as a side dish or include it in your morning smoothie.

Non-Stop Paleohack 2.0: Throw out your nonstick skillet, as it is very toxic. Simply use a stainless-steel skillet and plenty of coconut oil when making omelets or scrambled eggs.

Lunch and Dinner
Staple Ingredients
Vegetables

- Cauliflower
- Asparagus
- Broccoli
- Tomatoes
- Sweet potatoes
- Yams
- Onions
- Lettuce and greens
- Spinach
- Carrots
- Bell peppers
- Other mixed greens, such as kale, arugula, and swiss chard
- Herbs and spices
- Cucumbers

Protein
Always try to buy organic and grass-fed meats as well as wild-caught ocean seafood.

- Beef
- Chicken
- Lamb
- Egg whites from free-range chickens
- Salmon and other fatty fish
- Bison

Healthy Fats

- Avocados
- Olives
- Walnuts
- Olive oil
- Almonds
- Macadamia nuts
- Salmon and other ocean-raised fatty fish
- Grass-fed beef and bison
- Organic egg yolks from free-range chickens
- Coconut oil

Non-Stop Paleo Lunch and Dinner Meals

- Grilled chicken breast with side salad and sweet potato fries
- Naked bison burger topped with tomatoes, avocado slices, and onions and served with roasted carrots
- Roasted spaghetti squash with red sauce
- Grilled salmon served with cauliflower mashed potatoes
- Taco salad made with beef, served over mixed kale and spinach, tomatoes, onions, red bell peppers, and avocados

- Roasted chicken served with steamed broccoli and a side salad
- Stir-fry, with your favorite vegetables and chopped protein in coconut oil
- Cheeseless pizza made from an almond flour crust, with any Paleo toppings of your choice
- Shrimp kebabs served on a mixed salad with olive oil and vinegar

Sides

- Sweet potato fries
- Cauliflower rice
- Roasted brussels sprouts drizzled with balsamic vinegar
- Beet salad served with chopped red onions and dressed with olive oil and red wine vinegar
- Roasted cauliflower seasoned with garlic salt and butter from grass-fed animals
- Baked sweet potatoes with scallions and butter from grass-fed animals
- Grilled artichokes drizzled with lemon juice, salt, and pepper
- Steamed or lightly sautéed asparagus topped with olive oil and lemon

As you can see, the *Non-Stop Paleo Diet* basically consists of a lean, healthy protein (yum) served with different types of salads and other roasted, grilled, steamed, or raw vegetables.

If you have to ask, it is probably not paleo.
—Robb Wolf

Snacks

There are plenty of healthy Paleo treats and snacks you can buy and also bake. If you simply Google "paleo baking" or "paleo cookies" for example, you will find thousands of options for fun, healthy, and great-tasting snacks you can prepare at home. I also have plenty of delicious recipes (as well as sample meals) at my website, www. NonStopPaleo.com.

I didn't intend this book to be a cookbook, so I am not going to go into depth about Paleo recipes, but I did want to give you an idea of what to reach for on your work break as well as weekend game snacks and healthy options for your children throughout the day. Always be prepared with some of these ideas at home and at work so you don't reach for an unhealthy option.

Healthy Options

- Dark chocolate
- Kale chips
- Trail mix
- Roasted and salted almonds (always use sea salt)
- Pistachios
- Sunflower seeds
- Fresh berries
- Guacamole
- Beef jerky
- Paleo granola
- Smoked salmon
- High-quality pepperoni, salami, or chorizo
- Veggies and hummus
- Mixed olives
- Pickles
- Veggie sticks with almond butter

Also check out chapter 9 for my latest and greatest Paleohacks, to find out how easy it is to eat Paleo meals and Paleo snacks and cook with everything Paleo. Again, *Non-Stop Paleo* is meant to keep your life exciting, palatable, and extremely healthy for the entire family, so you have the desire to continue this healthy journey for your entire life!

To be honest with you, once you get the food and ingredients down, all else falls into place, and it will be easy for you to keep going because you will feel so good. If you do happen to fall off the wagon after following the guidelines laid out in this book, you will feel so crappy that you will remember why you started *Non-Stop Paleo* in the first place.

Action Steps

- Put together a grocery list of the items in this chapter, go to your local health-food store, and purchase the essential Paleo ingredients.
- Purchase a few Paleo cookbooks to get more meal and snack ideas.
- Follow my Paleo blog for more Paleo meals, snacks, and recipes at http://www.nonstoppaleo.com/category/nonstoppaleo-recipes/.
- On Sunday nights, write out and plan your weekly meals and snacks for the next seven days. (Remember to put in your cheat meal too.)
- Also on Sundays, feel free to do any food-prep work that will make your week go easier and keep you on track.
- Always have healthy Paleo snacks on hand to keep you on track in the beginning or during stressful times.

CHAPTER 4

Living the Non-Stop Paleo Way

*People who think "going paleo" is just
about food and diet choices are missing
the boat. Going Paleo is an entire lifestyle
that affects all your decision making.*
—Dr. Nick Caras

As I mentioned above, once you get the *Non-Stop Paleo* ingredients, foods, and meal-planning down, you will be able to dive into other aspects of your life with regard to how our Paleolithic ancestors lived. This is where most people go wrong. They can start to eat healthier, but everything else in their life is not as Paleo as it should be. Do you ever wonder why, when you start a new diet and/or exercise program, the weight doesn't seem to come off? We have to start to take this *Paleo way of life* to our entire daily routine, not just some new food choices.

Have you ever wondered how our ancestors exercised? Were they under extreme amounts of stress and worries? Did they have bills to pay, financial worries, office stress, traffic, a household in disarray, and so forth? Did they go hit the treadmill for forty-five minutes a day with a nice, slow jog? Were they stuck inside all day, or did they actually get outside and get some sunlight? Do you think our older generations were exposed to all the environmental toxins, household-cleaning toxins, and various toxic materials that are found in our bathroom products, such as deodorants, toothpastes, soaps, shampoos, makeup, lotions, and much more?

I hope you get the picture here. It's not just about the unhealthy food that plagues our world today. So much has changed in just a few generations, let alone hundreds or thousands of years. We live in a much different world than our ancestors did. Don't get me wrong; I love the technology and conveniences just as much as you do, but there are steps we can take to minimize the detrimental effects that living in this century affords us.

My favorite part of being in private practice and helping so many people is that I get to hack their entire lifestyles, not just their diets. Through patient consultations and patient education, I am able to teach individuals, parents, and families how to rearrange their lifestyles within this world of conveniences and technology. Really, all you have to do is make some minor changes that will seem quite easy after I explain them to you. Again, once you implement them, you will notice the health benefits almost immediately and will love the way you look, feel, and function. Your overall health will increase with regard to your energy levels, immune system, mood, and so much more going on at the cellular level. This is the missing piece in modern health care. So, where should we begin? How about your exercise routine?

Non-Stop Paleo Exercise

I have great news for you. The days of spending an hour or more in the gym each and every day are long gone. The days of lacing up the running shoes and going out for a ten-mile jog that literally takes up your whole morning are long gone, too! You no longer have to plan your whole day around your exercise routine. Our ancestors never exercised this way and neither should you. It is too time-consuming, and it's actually DETRIMENTAL to your health. It is time to start exercising the way that is actually BENEFICIAL to your health, weight-loss goals, immune system, and longevity!

Since the 1960s we have been on a cardiovascular craze. Yes, I believe cardiovascular health is important, but we have been going about it all wrong. We have been wasting time, energy, and health with the way we work out and continue to exercise.

Are you still under the impression that long-distance training is beneficial for your heart, lungs, blood vessels, and weight loss? Well, with the new information you will find in these pages, you are going to say good-bye to those worn-out treadmills and running shoes. It's time to get you a new pair of cross-trainers. No more thirty- to sixty-minute jogs, bikes, or elliptical machines. You no longer have to wake up two hours before the sun comes up because you have to go get a ten- or fifteen-mile jog in.

Long-distance training has never really been beneficial to your heart or longevity—in fact, quite the opposite. You see, long-distance training of any kind is actually hurting you. It puts way too much pressure on your body at the cellular level. Research has shown that running a marathon can cause irreversible damage each time you participate in one, and all the training runs and long-distance runs you do add up to cellular damage on your body as well.

The goal of the *Non-Stop Paleo Life* is to keep you healthy through each generation of life so that you can age gracefully and enjoy life to the fullest both physically and mentally. The burden that long-distance cardiovascular training puts on your body wears your entire body down and ages you quicker. I have seen thousands of patients with worn-down joints due to activities such as long-distance biking and running. They can live with this discomfort in their thirties and forties, but when they get into their fifties, sixties, and beyond, they tend to be in a lot of pain and discomfort. This is no way to live. This is not aging gracefully. They are forced to alter their lifestyles and hobbies due to their pain and discomfort.

What is the *Non-Stop Paleo* way to exercise? Well, our Paleolithic ancestors didn't exercise per se, but they were moving and living high-intensity lifestyles. This is where High-Intensity Interval Training (HIIT) came from. Since they lived this way, it is still engrained in our DNA to this very day. You see, our DNA actually hasn't changed much since the Paleolithic Era, which is another good reason to go Paleo in all aspects of life. What was good for the health of people in that era is still good for our health today!

Again, they didn't really exercise for the sake of exercising, but they were moving, hiking, climbing, running after food, sprinting from predators, and the like. Such movements make up the essence of cross-training and HIIT. How does *Non-Stop Paleo* exercise look like in 2017?

We do not have to sprint from predators, run after our food, or climb and hike all day long to gather our next meal, but we still need to incorporate the corresponding movements into our lifestyles. There are many different ways to do HIIT in today's world. In fact, most cardio machines at your local gym already have this training protocol programmed in for you. This is the one where you do a very high-intensity sprint for one minute and then a walk-out or cool-down for the next minute. Do this for a short twenty minutes, and you will be worn out and dripping in sweat. This is all it really takes to get a great cardio workout in just twenty minutes a day every other day!

This is just one form of interval cardio training. There are all different types of boot camps, spin classes, cross-training programs, cross-fit gyms, and stair-climbing groups, among others. The list is endless; whichever form of cardio you prefer can be turned into HIIT.

Sample Twenty-Minute HIIT Workout

Week	Reps	Work: Hill Sprints (Seconds)	Recovery: Walk-Backs (Minutes)	Total Time (Minutes)
1	6	60	2	18
2	8	60	2	24
3	10	60	1.5	25
4	10	45	1.5	22.5

On your off days, some form of resistance training should be done. Whether you like to hit the weights, the machines, or body-weight exercises like pull-ups and push-ups, resistance training is a key part of staying Paleo. Do not overthink weight training or get too scientific with it. Just make sure you are working each body part at least once a week.

The other form of exercise that our Paleolithic ancestors got in each day was simply walking. Do not underestimate the power of walking. The human DNA was never meant to sit all day long as we do now. Our children sit in school and then hit the couch for video games and television; we adults sit at desks, in cars, and on couches most of their lives. Sitting adds up and is very detrimental to your health and longevity.

> *Sitting will soon be considered the "new smoking." I believe it is seriously that detrimental to your overall health and well-being.*
> *—Dr. Nick Caras*

It is time we understood that we can no longer sit all day and think we can be healthy. Fortunately, there are many tips and tricks you can do to get by. For starters, go for a walk after dinner each night instead of grabbing the remote. On your coffee breaks at work, go outside, breathe some fresh air, and walk around your office building once or twice. Invest in a stand-up desk or, better yet, a treadmill desk. Try taking the stairs every once in a while. Just keep moving and walking throughout the day. If you're on the phone a lot, get a headset and stay on your feet while you're talking. It is actually pretty easy once you set your mind to moving throughout the day. This should be one of your simplest Paleo strategies to implement tomorrow. Purchase a Fitbit to track your daily steps. Our Paleo ancestors got in over twenty thousand steps every day. You should strive for at least ten thousand steps per day, not including your exercise.

Non-Stop Paleo Detoxification

Did our Paleolithic ancestors do regular detoxes, cleanses, colon flushes, and the like? Of course they didn't. My patients always ask me, "How can I include detoxification in anything Paleo when they didn't detoxify during that time frame?" The answer is simple: They didn't detox because they didn't have to. All the common toxins that surround us today were not around during the Paleolithic Era.

We are completely surrounded by chemical toxins. There is no getting around it. They are everywhere: in our food chain; on our furniture, carpets, and mattresses; in cleaning supplies, laundry detergent, and dish soap; and in the bathroom cabinet in the form of toothpaste, deodorant, soaps, and shampoos. Toxins are in the air that we breathe and the water that we drink. No matter how clean we think we are living, our bodies are going to be bombarded with chemical toxins on a daily basis. These toxins will build up in our organs, tissues, and cells and eventually wear different parts of our bodies down, age us quicker than normal, and even cause disease.

It is not up for debate whether we should detoxify on a regular basis or not. The answer is a resounding yes; as a matter of fact, I believe you should start tomorrow.

Inside each cell of the body are little molecular structures called mitochondria. The job of the mitochondria is to produce energy. The more efficient your mitochondria are working, the healthier you can be. One of the main reasons toxins are so harmful to you is that toxins will wear down the efficiency of your mitochondria, thus making your entire body much less efficient.

If we can support the natural detoxification protocols of your body, your mitochondria will work much more efficiently, which will allow you to be much healthier for years to come. So how should you go about detoxifying? Before I dive into that, I want to let you know that there is a big difference between cleansing your body and detoxifying it.

I am sure you've heard of a water cleanse or lemon-water cleanse, during which you might only drink lemon water for twenty-four or forty-eight hours straight and not consume any food or other drinks. I want you to think of a cleanse as just giving your body a break—giving your stomach, digestive tract, colon, liver, and kidneys a break from processing your daily food (and the toxins that come with it). Although a cleanse is healthy and the much-needed break is appreciated by your internal organs, it is not a detox. A detox is just what it sounds like: the excretion of harmful toxins from your body.

The solution to pollution is dilution.
—Dr. Bob Rakowski

We named the aforementioned substances *toxins* because they are poisons that are very hard to excrete from your body. A classic example of a toxin is mercury, which is very harmful to your brain, nervous system, and other organs. Mercury is probably in your body right now, and you should do everything you can to detox it out.

First and foremost, try to eliminate toxins from your food and your home by living as green and clean as possible. Then try some of my favorite ways to detoxify your body:

- Pharmaceutical-grade supplements and detox shakes
  - Vitamin C
  - Milk Thistle
  - Selenium
  - Magnesium
  - Alpha-Linoleic Acid
  - Methionine
  - Methylated folic acid
  - CoQ10
  - Acetyl-L-Carnitine
  - N-Acetyl Cysteine

- Increasing your body's Glutathione levels
    o   Undenatured whey protein
    o   N-Acetyl Cysteine
- Sweating, through daily HIIT exercise and infrared saunas
- Drinking more tea
- Eating organic
- Filtering your home's water by reverse osmosis
- Regular coffee enemas
- Exfoliating your skin
- Losing weight (Fat cells are a magnet for toxins.)

Non-Stop Paleo Thinking

This is the most overlooked part of your own personal health-care (self-care) system. You have to nail this one in order to be completely healthy and live a long, happy life. *Non-Stop Paleo Thinking* involves techniques you can use on a daily basis to keep you in a positive frame of mind throughout your busy, stressful life.

Did our Paleolithic ancestors use the techniques I am going to teach you? Probably not, but they did live with a sense of community that kept them engaged with each other, and they also did not live in a fast-paced world with thousands of daily stresses bombarding them each day. There were no e-mail in-boxes filled with negative messages or TV commercials constantly pushing a new pharmaceutical drug for yet another seemingly made-up disease. They didn't live paycheck to paycheck, and they were not living in fear as a lot of us are today. In the face of all these factors, I personally believe that adding in some healthy habits, which are outlined below, will make a tremendous difference in your life with regard to happiness, wellness, productivity, and success.

Trust me, everyone—your children, your spouse, coworkers, siblings, and parents—will benefit from these techniques. You will not have to use all the techniques and habits outlined below, but you should find out which ones resonate with you and start adding them to your daily routine. These techniques will work most effectively if you use them first thing in the morning and/or right before bed. It is time to train your brain for success. In order to make *Non-Stop Paleo* work for a lifetime, you must have a trained brain to keep you on track with your goals and wishes! Whether or not you will actually stick with this program or any new diet program largely depends on your mind-set.

*All our dreams can come true if we have
the courage to pursue them.
—Walt Disney*

Almost all of us can do any new program for two to four weeks. Big Deal—we are talking about the rest of your life here. Did you ever start a new program and stay hyped up about it for a few weeks? All of a sudden, though, you fell off the wagon because you had a weekend party to attend. From that point, the whole program spiraled down-ward, and you just couldn't or wouldn't put forth the work and energy it would take to get back onboard. We have all been there. It's called *yo-yo dieting.* Fad diets come and go and never last because they do not incorporate lifestyle programs that people can stick with. And they are almost ALWAYS missing the key ingredient: the way you **think**—for the long-term. Motivation should not be simply about a few weeks; it should be for the rest of your life. You have to start "thinking" the *Non-Stop Paleo way* today.

Below is a bunch of strategies you can start to implement today that will keep you in the right state of mind. Pick the habits and strate-gies that resonate with you, and put them in your daily routine. I firmly believe that acting on them in the morning is best. Getting yourself in the right mind-set each morning will set your brain up for success. You will be much more likely to stick with any program or accomplish any goal if you get yourself in the right mind-set as soon as you wake up.

Grateful Mind-Set

Having a grateful mind-set is the number-one way to stay positive. Just look around: there are plenty of things to be grateful and thankful for. The strategy here is to keep a journal by your bedside. As soon as you wake up, grab your journal and your pen and write down a few things that you are grateful for. Do this exercise before bed as well. If you put your brain in a grateful mind-set, it cannot be in an angry or depressed mood. It is as simple as that. All day long you are going to be bombarded with negative thoughts and emotions and stressful situations; it is essential that you keep yourself in a grateful mind-set as opposed to an anxious or stressed-out mind-set.

Visualization

Many of us are visual learners or visual people. We like to see things. Visualization can go hand in hand with goal-setting. Get pictures of your goals, and put them on your bathroom mirror or some other place where you can look at them each day. Take time to look at these pictures and go over your goals. Whether it is healthy food, certain exercises, better finances, happy children, or being able to fit into a new bikini, get pictures of all these things so you can see them each morning. This will stimulate your brain to stay on track. You will be much less likely to fall off the wagon at lunchtime if your brain and visual cortex have been stimulated by your positive visualizations each morning. Some people make entire vision boards that they hang somewhere in their homes. This is another great strategy. As your goals change, your visions should change as well. Always be updating your pictures and vision boards with new goals, new ideas, and other things that make you happy and put you in the right mind-set.

Prayer or Meditation

A lot of my patients like to use prayer or meditation to keep them on track. This is a great strategy as it can stimulate your conscious and unconscious brain. It doesn't matter what religion or belief system you happen to practice. When you get your mind and body into a deep, relaxed state of mind, you are actually training your brain to stay on course. With the help of this habit, as well as the others, you are likely to stay on track with your goal and much less likely to cheat or fall off the wagon. People who practice meditation on a regular basis are some of the most successful people in the world.

> *Meditation is a way to let the noise settle and see what's inside.*
> *—Russell Simmons*

Journaling

Writing is another strategy that stimulates your brain and puts you in a great frame of mind. Writing down your thoughts, goals, fears, and accomplishments can help put your body and mind at ease and let stresses melt away. Journaling is a great tool to do right before bed and first thing upon waking. Getting things off your chest right before bed will help you sleep much deeper. With better sleep comes a healthier and more rejuvenated body that could lead you to automatically start to make healthier choices in your daily life. By journaling first thing in the morning, you are setting up your day for success. You will accomplish more, feel better about yourself, and become a much more successful person both personally and professionally.

These are a few techniques I personally like to use, and I highly recommend them to you. There are many other techniques out there as well, but the bottom line is you MUST practice something each day. If not, you are more than likely to fall off the wagon at some point.

I came up with the *Non-Stop Paleo Program* because I envisioned a *Non-Stop* healthy way of life for people. I was so sick of motivating people for a couple weeks or a month and watching them see and feel their results only to watch them fall right back into their same old ruts. After another couple of months, they find themselves back in my office with the same old symptoms.

After years of frustration and wondering why people couldn't stick with a program, I discovered the common denominator and came up with the missing ingredient—*Non-Stop Paleo Thinking*!

Here are some other techniques and strategies that might resonate with you. Choose the ones that work for you and make them a part of your morning routine, just like brushing your teeth each morning. It is vital for you to develop a positive mind-set.

- Goal-setting
- Quiet thinking time
- Meditation
- Visualization and vision boards
- Planning and Journaling
- Slow-breathing techniques
- Yoga
- Being grateful
- Reading
- Walking
- Stretching

Action Steps

- Commit to HIIT training instead of long-distance training.
- Plan and write down your exercise routine with regard to cardio, resistance training, and core training. Know exactly which days you are going to be performing the different forms of exercise needed to stay Paleo.
- Get a Fitbit (or similar device) to track your daily steps. Strive for at least twenty thousand steps per day.

- Throw out all your household chemical toxins, and replace them with clean-living supplies such as essential oils and vinegar.
- Start to eat more organic foods and non-GMO (genetically modified organism) foods whenever possible.
- Start to detoxify your body on a regular basis. Daily, weekly, and monthly detox protocols are essential to longevity.
- Write out your goals and visions for the year.
- Make a Vision Board and place it somewhere you will see it every day (such as on the bathroom mirror).
- Start to journal each night before bed and first thing in the morning.
- Take the grateful challenge: write out a few things you are grateful for each morning.
- Start yoga, Pilates, walking, or stretching each morning while practicing your visualizations.

CHAPTER 5

Does Your Health Insurance or Pharmacy Care about You?

*Your body's innate ability to heal itself is
more powerful than we will ever know.
—Dr. Nick Caras*

Who is in charge of your health? Who is accountable for how healthy, happy, and wonderful your life can be? Does your health-insurance carrier call you in the morning to ask how you're feeling? Does the local pharmacy or pharmaceutical representative ever ask you how that medicine is doing and if you are feeling better since taking it?

I have news for you: there is only one person in charge of your health—YOU! As a society, we rely on others to take care of our health. Our doctors (medical and alternative), our drugs, our pharmacies, our physician's assistants, and even our DNA often get the blame if we are not feeling well, are sick, or have some nasty disease. It is time for us to look in the mirror. By the way, since we are in control of our genes, we cannot blame them or let others blame our genes either. Blaming your inheritance is a scapegoat answer that will keep you in the unhealthy lifestyle you have become accustomed to.

I'll say it again: it is time for us to look in the mirror and take all the blame for how healthy or unhealthy we currently are. How many times in your life have you switched insurance? Every time you get a new job, you most likely get a new insurance plan and carrier. Sometimes they pay for certain treatments and tests, and other times they do not. The only constant about insurance companies is that they will keep making money. They will always accept monthly premiums, but when you need a certain treatment or test, they are not always there for you. Sometimes they don't even pay your medical doctor, and the bill is left to you. Unfortunately, that is just the way it is, and it is only getting worse.

It is not my intention to bash insurance companies, be they private or federal. I do not want to field questions about the United States moving toward a socialized health-care system. There is no one-size-fits-all system that will save the country or make us all healthy again. The answer lies with you. It always has, and it always will. The CEOs of health-insurance carriers are not sitting at home right now wondering how you are feeling. There may be a way to fix the US health-care system, but it is going to be an uphill battle. Fortunately for you, you have taken a great first step by buying this book and learning its tools and strategies to make you and your family healthy.

You have to care about You. Take care of your health. Live by the 90/10 rule with regard to the healthy habits and lifestyle changes you are learning about in this book. Start today! When we quit blaming others, for example, our doctors, our drugs, and our health-insurance companies, we will all become empowered to be as healthy as we possibly can be.

I am a firm believer that you must continue to read, research, study, and learn about the Paleo lifestyle and what it takes to be healthy for a lifetime. Commit to your new lifestyle, watch your weight loss improve and your energy levels and happiness increase, and you'll end up wondering why you didn't get the flu or a cold this year. Start the strategies and tips you will learn in this book with your entire family. If you are single, start this new lifestyle with friends, neighbors, and coworkers. You will be much more successful that way. Make it fun. Again, it is up to you to start making healthy decisions. Lucky for you, in chapter 9 I have laid out many Paleohacks to make your life much easier with regard to making the right choices—the healthy choices—day in and day out.

The one thing you cannot do is continue to blame outside sources for your current health. Accept where your current level of health is, and start to move forward.

Action Steps

- Take a stand for your health, and fill in the blanks:

    I do not blame_____ for my current
        level of health.
    I do not blame_____ for my current
        level of health.
    I do not blame_____ for my current
        level of health.
    I do not blame_____ for my current
        level of health.
    I do not blame_____ for my current
        level of health.
    Who is responsible for your health?_____

- Understand that every decision you make today moves you either closer to health or closer to sickness and disease.
- Start making healthier choices in every aspect of your life.
- Make a morning affirmation, stating that you are in control of your DNA, your life, your current situation, and your overall picture of health. For example:

Today, I am in control of my decisions and will make healthy decisions with regards to exercise, food choices, happiness levels, and overall stress levels. This empowers me to be in control of my own health and well-being. Nobody else can determine how healthy I am going to be today. Today I declare to live life to the fullest, knowing that I am in control.

CHAPTER 6
Blood Tests and Supplementation

Blood Tests

For a doctor in private practice, there is no better snapshot of someone's health than blood work. I love getting some very specific blood tests done to help me determine where a patient's health is and what direction I need to move the patient in. The blood work that I do for my patients is probably going to sound a little different from what you are used to. I want to show you what I look at and why.

Without a starting point like blood work, determining a treatment plan to move forward with would be just a guessing game. Below is a list of tests I like to run, with a brief description of the information I am trying to get from them. My concern is for getting an overall picture as to where the patient is right now, health wise.

Vitamin D

Get your vitamin D tested today! You need to know your number. Out of all the blood work that can possibly be ordered, vitamin D is at the top of my list. This is because vitamin D really isn't even a vitamin; it is a hormone, and it regulates many systems and processes in your body.

In fact, one great piece of research shows that increased vitamin-D levels in your body reduce all causes of morbidity. It is that important.

Another great reason you need to know your vitamin D is that it is huge in fighting cancer. One in two Americans are now going to get cancer. It is not a matter of *if*; it is a matter of *when*. Why not take this easy vitamin on a daily basis to ensure your D levels are high and that your body is naturally fighting cancer day in and day out?

> *Vitamin D is a steroid hormone that influences virtually every cell in your body. Low levels are linked to poor bone health, as well as heart, brain, immune, and metabolic dysfunction.*
> *—Dr. Mercola*

I always get the question, "What should my vitamin D number be?" It is very confusing because the so-called acceptable range in the United States is so wide. Currently a recommended vitamin-D level falls between thirty and ninety-nine. This is a complete joke in my mind; I believe that research shows that we need to be at a minimum of sixty. I actually encourage my patients to stay above seventy-five. When your vitamin D is up at these levels, your immune system can function properly. Not only will you get fewer colds, flus, and other sicknesses, but you will be combatting cancer and other deadly diseases.

Unfortunately, I commonly see vitamin-D levels below twenty. It is very unfortunate, because I know that people at that level are on the verge of a health crisis and must make changes immediately. The natural way to get vitamin D is from the sun. The problem is that most of us do not spend enough time in the sun, and when we do, we put on sunscreen that protects us in one way but also blocks vitamin-D absorption. In the Paleolithic Era, people didn't have this issue; they spent a lot of time in the sun and were able to get proper vitamin-D absorption. Everyone, children as well as adults, should be supplementing with vitamin-D levels until proven otherwise by blood work.

HgA1c

Over the past decade, the United States has finally caught up to research, and we now know that sugar is behind almost all chronic diseases. In my mind, your sugar levels are among the most important factors you need to get under control. Diabetes and prediabetes are crucial risk factors in many disease processes. If you want to live a long, vibrant, and healthy life, your sugar levels have to be in check.

How do we check sugar levels? Well, some practitioners use a glucose test, but this can be misleading; sometimes, we can trick a simple glucose blood test by fasting for twelve hours the day before the test. This may make our glucose test look good, and we can go on feeling good about ourselves and start eating a bad diet again. An improved test is the HgA1c or Hemoglobin A1C. Think of a HgA1c test as a three-month average of the sugar levels in your bloodstream. The HgA1c test is something that cannot be cheated. I will know if patients are lying about their diets because HgA1c is giving me a longer look at their sugar levels.

I cannot stress enough how bad sugar, too much fructose, and processed foods are for our health and longevity. The *Non-Stop Paleo Lifestyle* eliminates so many of these bad foods that your sugar consumption will automatically go down. We need to remember that Paleolithic people did not have inflammation and/or sugar-regulation problems. This is why their incidences of heart disease and cancer were so low. Next time you are at your doctor's office for blood work, make sure to request the HgA1c test so you can make a conscious decision on your sugar intake going forward.

Omega-6/3 Ratio

This is another vital piece of blood work that I personally run on myself and my family each year. Let's start with a little bit of background about omegas. Omega-3s are the healthy anti-inflammatory omegas, while omega-6s are the very unhealthy pro-inflammatory omegas. Both are fats, but there is a very distinct difference between good fats and bad fats. We are meant to eat a lot of good fats in each meal, and we were never meant to eat any bad fats. Below are lists of good fats versus bad fats from food sources.

Good Fats	Bad Fats
Avocados	Sunflower oil
Olives	Conventionally raised meats
Coconut oil	Trans fats
Grass-fed butter	Soybean oil
Egg yolks	Fried foods
Grass-fed meats	Corn oil
Nuts	Margarine
Seeds	Safflower oil
Olive oil	Pastries and other packaged goods
Fish-oil supplements	

Supplementation with good fats is also a must. We should get these additional good fats from fish-oil supplementation. If you are taking fish-oil vitamins and staying away from all the bad omega-6 fats, you will be able to keep your omega-6s to omega-3s very close to a one-to-one ratio in your bloodstream. This is the ratio you want; it will ensure that you maintain your body in an anti-inflammatory state. As we know, inflammation is one of the underlying factors in almost all sicknesses and diseases. Right now, most Americans are not even close to a one-to-one ratio. Most are at twenty-to-one or higher, which means that they are very inflamed.

So, to reiterate, there are two ways to get your ratio in range. One way is to start taking fish-oil supplements and eating healthy fats in your diet, which will improve the omega-3s in your body. The other is to quit eating the bad fats or omega-6 fats listed above. By following the *Non-Stop Paleo Diet*, you will not be consuming omega-6 fats, for the most part. It is truly a shame that the US government actually recommends eating omega-6 fats like vegetable oil and other grains in the first place. It has caused so much inflammation and disease in this country. Quit eating this junk immediately. Not quitting would be one of the most detrimental things you could do to your health.

CRP

C-Reactive Protein, or CRP for short, is another great tool we have to measure inflammation. I suggest that my patients and clients get to know their CRP levels. As an indicator of silent inflammation, it also assesses your chances of developing heart disease and/or cancer, the two biggest killers in the United States. If we take a proactive role and learn our inflammation levels, we can seriously decrease our chances of being struck by these two major diseases. When lifestyle factors such as smoking, obesity, decreased exercise/activity, and having diabetes are present, levels of CRP will naturally rise in the body. This is no surprise as these are also factors in heart disease and cancer.

It is good to test your CRP levels on a regular basis (every year or two) in order to keep you motivated in your lifestyle choices and the *Non-Stop Paleo* routine. When we are not proactive and do not know our numbers, it is very easy to fall off the wagon. CRP is a much better indicator than cholesterol for all forms of heart disease. I will not go into depth in this book about what I call the cholesterol "hoax" (that will be for the next book), but I will say that you can quit worrying about cholesterol; it's a bad indicator of heart disease, whereas your CRP levels are much better indicators. Get to know your numbers and, if you are high, adopting the *Non-Stop Paleo Lifestyle* should get your numbers down into range.

Food Allergy

This isn't the more common testing that an allergist would perform. Food allergies basically show up in two different ways. The one most of us think about is called IgE (Immunoglobulin E) allergies. This is when someone who is allergic to shellfish, for example, accidentally eats a lobster and has an immediate reaction. The person may break out into hives, have trouble breathing, or even go into anaphylactic shock. Although these food reactions are very serious, they are not what I am concerned with in this book. By the time most patients walk into my office, they already know if they have a shellfish, peanut, or similar allergy.

The food-allergy testing I would like to shed some light onto is for *IgG* (Immunoglobulin G) allergies. If you have an IgG reaction to a particular food, you will not even know it unless you ever have the blood work done. It is a very subtle reaction, such that your body can actually have an inflammatory response to that food at any time in the ensuing forty-eight hours. It is not an immediate response.

These reactions can cause symptoms like headaches (including migraines), acne, psoriasis, bloating, digestive issues, hyperactivity, and leaky-gut syndrome (described in "Probiotics," below).

This is the single best test to do when a patient has tried just about everything but cannot seem to get better. Patients in this situation may find out they are allergic to something considered extremely healthy—apples, perhaps—and that their rare allergies have been triggering their migraines. They would have never known or ever guessed that eating apples was the problem because the food doesn't cause the headaches until two days later.

IgG food-allergy testing is so simple and easy that I believe everyone should have it done. We are all individuals, and the only way we will really know what foods to eat will come from our own individual blood work. Once you eliminate foods that are causing inflammatory reactions in your body, your entire immune system will likely grow much stronger. It will work more efficiently and have more time to fight stuff like bacteria, viruses, and cancer cells instead of just the foods it doesn't like.

Vitamins and Other Supplementation

Nearly all disease can be traced to a nutritional deficiency.
—Dr. Linus Pauling, two-time Nobel Prize winner

Fish Oil

Fish oil contains a couple of the healthy fats called omega-3s. These fats are essential to human function for a variety of reasons. Most importantly, they are anti-inflammatory! As you may have noticed by now, most people are eating and living in a very INFLAMMATORY way. Since we know that inflammation is the root of all diseases and lifestyle conditions, it is very important to take fish oil to help offset inflammation levels. Once you adopt the *Non-Stop Paleo Diet*, you will be eating a much less inflammatory diet, but it is still essential to take a daily fish-oil supplement.

Do not be confused by companies that try to sell you omega-3s that are not from fish oil. The human body needs the omega-3s that you can only get from clean, healthy fish. Here is a list of health benefits that you receive from fish oil:

- Boosts the immune system
- Fights cancer
- Decreases chances of heart disease
- Aids in brain function
- Aids in brain and nervous-system development in children
- Decreases inflammation levels
- Helps stop "leaky gut"
- Enhances cellular communication
- Decreases anxiety and depression rates

Fish-supplementation will help with these specific conditions:

- Depression
- Cardiovascular disease
- Type II diabetes
- Fatigue
- Dry, itchy skin
- Brittle hair and nails
- Inability to concentrate
- Joint pain
- High blood pressure
- Anxiety
- ADD/ADHD
- Alzheimer's disease
- Asthma
- Excessive menstrual pain
- High cholesterol
- Osteoporosis
- Compromised immune system
- Fatigue
- Epilepsy
- For cancer patients, inability to maintain a healthy weight
- Rheumatoid arthritis
- Atherosclerosis
- Crohn's disease
- Ulcerative colitis
- Bipolar disorder

Be cautious of buying just any old fish-oil supplement from the market aisle. You should always get fish-oil supplements from your natural-health-care provider to ensure quality, cleanliness, and freshness of the oil. Since our oceans are highly polluted with mercury and other harsh toxins, so are the fish that live in the ocean. Make sure your fish-oil capsules have been molecularly distilled to ensure purity and cleanliness. Ask your health-care provider if your fish oil has been molecularly distilled. If it has not, find a brand that is so distilled. It is vital that you not consume mercury and other toxins each time you take your fish-oil supplement. This is even more important for your children with their developing brains and bodies.

For the best fish oil I have found on the market, check out my online vitamin store at http://drnick.metagenics.com/store. You can find pure, molecularly distilled fish oil here for adults and for children.

How to Get Essential Omega-3 Fats in Your Diet

Food Source	Serving Size	Grams of Omega-3
Cod-liver oil	1 tbs.	2.8
Walnuts	1 oz.	2.6
Mackerel	4 oz.	2.2
Flaxseeds	1 oz.	1.8
Sardines	4 oz.	1.8
Salmon	4 oz.	1.7
Swordfish	4 oz.	1.7
Scallops	4 oz.	0.5
Shrimp	4 oz.	0.37
Pecans	1 oz.	0.3
Broccoli	1 c.	0.2
Raspberries	1 c.	0.12
Spinach	½ c.	0.1
Kale	½ c.	0.1

Probiotics

Gut bacteria (intestinal flora) are the bacteria that line our intestinal tracts. These are good bacteria that perform many bodily functions.

Healthy microorganisms that reside in the intestines, such as the *Lactobacilli* species, form part of the body's defense system against food-borne pathogens and microorganisms. Without them, we could not survive. Don't get me wrong: there are definitely a lot of bad bacteria that we encounter every day through breathing, touching, and eating, but there are also millions of good bacteria inside our digestive tracts. We actually have around ten times the number of bacteria in our gut than we have cells in our entire body. These good bacteria inside us are big players in our immune systems. In order for us to have optimally functioning immune systems, we must have the right number of good bacteria lining our digestive tracts. With the proper number of good bacteria, we will have a much better chance of fighting off sickness and disease.

Over the past decade, there probably hasn't been a system of your body studied more in functional medicine than your gut. We are now finding out how much good *probiotic* bacteria are living inside your gut and digestive tract and how many different health benefits and functions these healthy probiotic bacteria perform. Mostly, your immune system is regulated by your gut bacteria. It is essential to keep replenishing your good bacteria on a daily basis.

There are basically two ways to make sure you have proper gut bacteria. You can and should eat and drink fermented foods with each meal or at least once each day, and you should also double down your bet and take a probiotic vitamin every single day. Your probiotic vitamin should have at least fifteen billion live organisms in each capsule.

If you do not keep up with the proper amount of good bacteria in your stomach and intestinal lining, you will start to develop *leaky-gut syndrome*, which occurs when your intestinal tract becomes weak and overtaken with bad bacteria, yeast, parasites, or fungi. You won't be able to digest your food properly or absorb nutrients properly. Toxins and other unhealthy substances will start to accumulate in your body.

Many people think that leaky-gut syndrome is a condition you either have or don't have. It's not really that black and white; there is a large gray area with this condition. In other words, we all probably have leaky gut to some extent; it is just a matter of how much. This is something we need to be aware of and constantly work on.

If you feel you have major digestive issues, including bloating, gas, constipation, and diarrhea, or if you just don't think you are absorbing nutrients properly and are constantly run-down or sick, check out these supplements to help get rid of your leaky gut:

- Probiotics
- Glutamine
- Digestive enzymes
- Fiber
- Prebiotics
- Fish oil

For more information on my personal, four-week, leaky-gut syndrome program, see http://www.nonstoppaleo.com/get-rid-of-leaky-gut/. This program will help get rid of leaky-gut syndrome fast and efficiently. But remember that it is not a black-and-white condition, so even after the four-week period, you still have to be diligent. Continue following the *Non-Stop Paleo* way of eating to keep your stomach and intestines functioning properly. This will also allow your good probiotic bacteria to flourish.

Vitamin D
As stated above (see "Blood Tests": "Vitamin D"), I cannot stress enough how important it is to keep your vitamin-D level within an optimal range (sixty minimum to eighty-five) to ensure your immune system is able to keep up with our fast-paced lifestyle.

Recall that in the Paleolithic times, people would normally get their vitamin D from the healthy UV-B rays from the sun. This is the natural way to get vitamin D. But we live and work inside most of the time and miss out on proper exposure from the midday sun. In addition, we have been brainwashed to coat on very toxic sunscreen that blocks the ability of the body to absorb vitamin D. Thus, our population's vitamin-D levels in general have fallen dramatically.

Since many of us do not get a lot of sun exposure and smartly cover up with sunscreen when we do go outside, vitamin D deficiency is common.
—Dr. Oz

In my **Paleo Lifestyle Eight-Week Bootcamp** (http://www.nonstop-paleo.com/paleo-lifestyle-8-week-bootcamp/), I have recommendations for how to get proper sun exposure without burning and for how to get enough vitamin D. If you are like most busy Americans, supplementing with vitamin D will likely be essential for your health.

Health Benefits of Vitamin D

- Boosts immune system
- Fights cancer
- Helps depression, anxiety, and other mental illnesses
- Helps maintain bone and muscle health
- Reduces diabetes risk
- Protects against cardiovascular disease
- Improves hormone function
- Helps fight the common cold, flu, and other infections

Whole-Food Multivitamin

This one is an obvious essential vitamin we need in our cupboard. A good multivitamin needs to be made from whole foods, not from synthetics (sound like the Non-Stop Paleo Life). A good multivitamin will not only contain everything from vitamin A to zinc but also whole-food superfoods and supernutrients.

Let's face it: most of us will never eat enough vegetables and whole foods to keep us at peak health in today's stressful world. Theoretically, even if you start to eat five pounds of broccoli with each meal, understand that the nutrient content of our vegetables today does not nearly compare to the nutrient content of vegetables twenty-five, fifty, and one hundred years ago, because our farming practices have depleted the soil of proper minerals and nutrients. Even if you adopt the *Non-Stop Paleo Lifestyle* and *Diet*, I urge you to hedge your bets and take a quality whole-food multivitamin to make sure your body is getting the vitamins, minerals, and other nutrients it needs all the way down to each individual cell.

Action Steps

- Find a health-care provider who has been trained in functional medicine and really cares about his or her patients.
- Make sure your new health-care provider knows about the specific blood tests I have outlined above. (Most functional-medicine doctors will routinely perform these types of tests.)
- Make sure your new health-care provider provides wellness, diet, and supplementation advice onsite.
- Start taking the essential vitamins and nutrients I have outlined above.
- Make sure you visit your functional-medicine doctor on a regular basis (as you would visit your dentist) to ensure that you are as healthy as you can be.

CHAPTER 7

Your Brain, Your Nervous System, and Why You Need Your Chiropractor

*I didn't know how much I could improve
until I started seeing a chiropractor. Since
I've been in chiropractic, I've improved
by leaps and bounds both mentally and
physically.*
—Michael Jordan

Some of the biggest misconceptions and areas of confusion in our entire health-care system are about chiropractic. Since 1895, when chiropractic was first discovered, it has been drastically underutilized by the American public. Even though it has completely changed people's lives, health, and well-being, it continues to be used as a Band-Aid™ modality for back and neck pain.

I would like to set the record straight on chiropractic. With only 7 percent of the American public utilizing chiropractic services, it is about time we start to understand what exactly chiropractic is, the science behind how and why it works, and why you and your family need to start seeing your local chiropractor on a regular basis. Just as you see your dentist for dental hygiene on a regular basis, you also need to see a chiropractor for brain, spine, and nervous-system hygiene on a regular basis.

Let's start with a little anatomy lesson. Your nervous system is the MOST IMPORTANT system in your body. It controls everything. Whether for a subconscious function like breathing or your heart beating, or a conscious decision like reaching your hand into the cupboard to grab a glass, your nervous system controls every cell, tissue, organ, and function in your body.

What exactly is your nervous system? Your nervous system is composed of three main parts: your brain, your spinal cord, and all the nerves that exit your spine and run through your entire body. Think of it as an electrical system. There is constant electrical flow coming down from your brain through your spinal cord and out to your body. Those electrical impulses that are flowing throughout your body are always regulating and controlling all the conscious and unconscious functions of your body.

So what does chiropractic medicine have to do with this? Well, as we go through our daily lives and come into contact with all sorts of stresses, this electrical system gets bombarded with static. Stress and static on the nervous system come in all forms. Some of the main stresses that you encounter in this day and age include posture issues, electromagnetic radiation from cell phones and Wi-Fi, sports injuries, car accidents and other traumas, pregnancy and then caring for your newborn and possibly other children, sitting all day long, overuse of muscles, and repetitive injuries. We are bombarded with all sorts of mental, physical, chemical, and emotional stresses all day long. Many of us find that there is not enough time in the day to accomplish everything we would like, and we all get overwhelmed from stress from time to time.

Your nervous system can only deal with so much stress before it starts to wear down a little bit. One of the first symptoms that you will feel when your nervous system starts to wear down is back pain, neck pain, and headaches. Some people will also feel fatigued, anxious, or depressed. This is exactly where chiropractic fits in and becomes so vital to your health.

The human body is a self-regulating organism, which means that it is programmed to heal itself. Pills will only mask your symptoms. The cure lies within yourself.
—Dr. Nick Caras

We all know that chiropractic is great at getting rid of your neck and back pain symptoms, but it is so much more than that. Chiropractic is actually a technique that revitalizes your nervous system and gets it functioning and firing back to 100 percent. This is what chiropractic was discovered for originally. It was never meant to be a modality like physical therapy. Chiropractic opens up the way your brain and body communicate. Without proper brain-to-body communication, your body starts to wear down and age at a much faster rate. Again, in order to continue to feel young, have proper flexibility and range of motion, and ensure proper nerve supply to your inside organs and tissues, you must make sure there is no static or impingement on your nervous system. Chiropractic spinal adjustments do just that.

Most people tend to wait until they are in pain before they see a chiropractor. This is why only 7 percent of the US population is utilizing chiropractic at any one time. Can you imagine if all of us received chiropractic adjustments just one time per month? We would all feel so much better! We would have more energy and a stronger immune system (fewer colds and flu symptoms) and feel younger and more vibrant. We would exercise better and, most importantly, we would age more gracefully and with less need for medication.

The country is now realizing that our health-care system is completely broken. Medications and surgeries will never be the answer for chronic lifestyle diseases. Our health-care system is now costing us so much money that it is on the way to bankrupting the United States. The time for change is right now. Do not fall victim to unnecessary medications and surgeries when there is a better way to live. Simply put, start to see your chiropractor on a more regular and preventive basis, and you too will reap the great health and longevity benefits that many others have discovered through chiropractic.

Action Steps

- Find a wellness-oriented chiropractor in your area.
- Start to receive wellness-chiropractic adjustments in order to make sure your brain-to-body connection is working properly.
- Share the chiropractic story with others so that everyone can benefit from a healthy nervous system and live a long, happy, and healthy life.

CHAPTER 8
Nutritional Ketosis

*Eat more FAT and be healthier than you
have been in years.
—Dr. Nick Caras*

Nutritional ketosis is a state in which your body efficiently burns
fat instead of sugar for energy. When you are able to turn your
body into a fat-burning machine, very good things start to
happen in your body.

It seems like everything we talk about always comes down to
sugar, and this is no different, but up until recently we always sought to
replace our sugar intake with protein. Research now suggests that this
is not the most beneficial way to go about your diet. Instead, replacing
sugar with healthy and high-quality fats may be much more beneficial
to the way you look and feel.

The term *ketogenic diet* is based on the name for certain molecules
in your body: *ketones*. Ketones are produced in your liver when no
sugar (glucose) is available for use. Glucose is one of the easiest substances for your body to use as fuel, so if there is sugar in your bloodstream because you just ate a bagel or drank some orange juice, then
your body will burn that sugar for energy. If your body cannot find any

sugar for fuel, then it has no choice but to start burning fat and using ketones as its primary energy source.

*Eating fat does not make you fat and
unhealthy; it is the sugar consumption!*
-Dr. Nick Caras

Once you have insulin resistance and sugar imbalances, your body goes into a downward spiral of inflammation, obesity, and fat-burning inefficiency. Now that sugar and insulin components have been identified in all chronic and degenerative lifestyle diseases, such as heart disease, most cancers, Alzheimer's and other dementias, arthritis, obesity, and mental disorders, among others, the ketogenic diet is coming to the forefront to combat diseases and slow down the aging process. By turning your body into a fat-burning machine (sending it into ketosis), the metabolic functions inside your brain, your liver, and every other cell in your body are going to act as if you are twenty-five years old again!

What exactly is the ketogenic diet? In short, the ketogenic diet is a HIGH-FAT, LOW-CARB, and LOW-PROTEIN diet. Your body will have no choice but to burn fat as fuel on this diet. It is very much like the Paleo diet but with a little less protein and a little less fruit, since fruit contains so much fructose, a sugar. Over and over again, research is suggesting that putting your body into ketosis can be the answer for all sorts of ailments and health issues.

Another benefit of the ketogenic diet is that your hunger cravings will go away very fast. By eating healthy fats, your body will get all the nutrition it needs and it will actually tell your brain that you are not hungry. Researchers have also found that you will most likely live longer when you are an efficient fat-burner (surprise, surprise). They have identified about a dozen genes connecting fat-burning and longevity!

How exactly do you get your body into a fat-burning ketotic state? The fastest and easiest way is to limit your net carbs per day while eating about 75 percent fat in your diet. Of course, this is fat from healthy sources (listed in chapter 3 and repeated below) and not trans fats or other unhealthy fats like canola or vegetable oils. Most research shows that you have to stay under fifty grams of net carbs per day, but I actually like a number around thirty grams of net carbs per day. This will then trigger your liver to start producing ketones, which tells us you are now burning fat as your primary fuel source and allowing the magic to start happening. You can test your ketone level very easily by a urine, blood, or even breath test. You can pick up a test kit over the counter at your local pharmacy and know exactly when your body is in ketosis. Nutritional ketosis is defined when your levels of ketones are within the range of 0.5–3.0 mmol/L (millimoles per liter).

OK, let's dive into the actual diet. What are you going to be eating on the ketogenic diet? First, let's go through a list of foods that I call "healthy fats." These foods are going to be around 75 percent of your diet, with the other 25 percent coming from protein and vegetables.

Healthy Fats

- Avocados
- Coconuts and coconut oil
- Olives and olive oil
- Eggs
- Grass-fed meats and poultry
- Fatty, wild-caught fish
  - Salmon
  - Snapper
  - Trout
  - Tuna
  - Mahi-mahi
  - Mackerel

- Almonds, walnuts, pecans, macadamias, and other nuts (excluding peanuts)
- Shellfish such as lobster, crabs, scallops, mussels, and clams
- Grass-fed bacon and sausage
- Organic and grass-fed butter

Sample Ketogenic Day
Breakfast
Three eggs (two whole eggs + one more egg yolk) scrambled in coconut oil and two slices of bacon.
Water, unsweetened tea, or Bulletproof Coffee (see below)

Lunch

Chicken lettuce wraps; using romaine lettuce for the wraps, fill with diced-up chicken breast, diced avocado, and diced tomato. Feel free to drizzle olive oil over the finished wrap.

Dinner

Naked burger topped with onion, lettuce, and avocado
Side salad

For an entire week's ketogenic diet, check out:
http://www.nonstoppaleo.com/ketogenic-diet-plan/

To reiterate, the ketogenic diet is very similar to the *Non-Stop Paleo Diet* but with less fruits and therefore a reduced net carb intake. Unlike the *Non-Stop Paleo Diet*, though, the ketogenic diet does not allow for cheat days; if you were to reintroduce sugar/additional carbs into your body, you would start to use those sugars instead of fat for energy, and you would no longer be in fat-burning mode.

A lot of you will notice that your body will actually be in nutritional ketosis by just following my *Non-Stop Paleo Diet*. I suggest you run out to your local pharmacy and get a test kit to help you to find out if and when you enter nutritional ketosis.

In my many years of research and private practice, I have observed patients who stay on a very low-carb, Paleo, and/or ketosis diet and look younger than their biological age, have much more energy, live longer, feel great, and do not really have any health problems like most Americans. Start fueling your body with 75 percent healthy fats, and you will see and feel the results almost immediately. Whether you are suffering from a chronic disease or you are a high-level athlete, the ketogenic diet will yield you the results you are looking for.

Action Steps

- Start incorporating at least 70 percent healthy fat with each meal.
- Purchase a ketone test kit from your local pharmacy and get into range (0.5–3.0 mmol/L).
- Consume a tablespoon of coconut oil two to three times per day.
- Purchase my week-long ketogenic diet and meal plan to get off on the right foot, at http://www.nonstoppaleo.com/ketogenic-diet-plan/.
- Start cooking your egg dishes with mostly the yolks, not the whites.
- Between meals, snack only on healthy fats like nuts, seeds, avocados, healthy jerky, olives, hard-boiled eggs, and smoked salmon.

- Drink Bulletproof Coffee first thing in the morning on an empty stomach (see chapter 9).
- Cook with only coconut oil.
- Start to drizzle olive oil on some of your dishes like salads, vegetables, omelettes, etc.

CHAPTER 9

Make It a Family Affair: Paleohacking and Biohacking in the Twenty-First Century

I have saved the best for last! This is my favorite chapter in the book. This is where I want to show you what we do in my household to keep my family of four extremely healthy in the fast-paced world we live in. Because we are all extremely busy and have spouses and children who depend on us and need us, sometimes healthy choices get pushed to the back burner in order to make life easier. Here I want to show you easy and affordable tips and tricks that you can start doing for yourself and your family.

In chapter 1, we touched upon biohacking, the practice of managing your own biology using nutritional, physical, or electronic techniques. Basically, it amounts to trying to get a positive health outcome in your body by experimenting with different methods. My goal has always been to use all-natural means to get to a state of complete health and wellness and to find out what works long-term for living a long, healthy life well into the hundreds.

In private practice, I have seen thousands of patients who have not aged so well. They are constantly sick, cannot get out of bed in the morning without medication, have no energy, and are chronically depressed or anxious. This is no way to live. Over the years, I have gathered information from these patients on how they lived their lives and why they think they have these conditions at the ages of sixty, seventy, eighty, and ninety. On the other hand, I have also treated eighty- and ninety-year-olds who look like they are sixty and still golf two times per week, swim, and enjoy life to the fullest. How can they be so happy, energetic, and full of life?

A better question might be, how do you want to feel and what do you want your life to be like when you are ninety or one hundred years old? Through talking to so many elderly people and listening to how they live their lives, and through biohacking my own body, I have compiled a list of strategies that you can start today that I believe will take your health to a much higher level!

I also coined the term *paleohacking* because many of these techniques fall right in line with the *Non-Stop Paleo Lifestyle*.

Here are my top paleohacks and other easy-to-implement strategies for the entire family.

1. Breakfast
2. Lunches and dinners
3. Kombucha tea
4. Fermented foods (vegetables)
5. Coconut
6. Bulletproof Coffee
7. Bone broth
8. Grass-fed meats
9. Walking every day
10. Avocados on everything
11. Olive-oil drizzling
12. Nuts and seeds
13. Cleaning the entire house with vinegar and water
14. Walking instead of watching TV
15. Egg yolk
16. Cave dwellers' sense of community

17. Getting off your Wi-Fi
18. Getting in the sun
19. Resistance training
20. Kale chips
21. Non-Stop Paleo Sleep
22. Fats
23. Turmeric
24. Starting each meal with a salad and/or veggies
25. Sprinting instead of jogging
26. Smoothies
27. Goals, affirmations, and journaling
28. Drinking nothing but water
29. Eating prior to work functions and other parties
30. Lemon or lime in your water
31. Saying NO to alcohol
32. Non-Stop Paleo pasta
33. Sprouting
34. Crockpots
35. Nontoxic mattresses
36. Intermittent fasting

Breakfast

On days or weeks when you are not participating in intermittent fasting (see paleohack 36, above), breakfast is probably your most important meal of the day. After making it this far in *The Non-Stop Paleo Life*, you most likely understand that most Americans' breakfast choices are very poor. Loaded with cereals, grains, gluten, sugar, and dairy, breakfast is like sending your brain and nervous system into a tornado before your day even gets going. No wonder kids cannot focus at school, are increasingly diagnosed with ADHD, and cannot finish projects. We are putting our brains in a hyperactive state before we go to school or work. What's the answer?

Well, for starters, throw out all your bread, toast, pancake mix, cereal boxes, and dairy milk and yogurt. Now we can get started. You want at least 50–70 percent of your breakfast calories to come from healthy fats. These healthy fats are what your body craves, and they will help your brain focus and work efficiently all the way to lunch time.

What should your food choices be? If you have time before you head out the door, I would suggest eggs. Eggs have been a SuperFood for centuries. Make sure you are buying and consuming "omega-3" eggs; conventionally raised chickens will typically produce omega-6 eggs. Remember, omega-3s are anti-inflammatory and extremely healthy, while omega-6s are the opposite. Contrary to popular belief, most of the health benefits of the egg are in the yolk. Make sure you are eating mostly yolks and a little bit of the whites. The ratio should be two yolks to every one white.

Just like you, I am in a rush most mornings to get a healthy meal to the kids and send them off to school before I head into the clinic. On such days, a healthy smoothie is a great option for breakfast.

A healthy smoothie should also contain great fats as well as organic fruits and vegetables. Here is a sample recipe I usually whip up in my Vitamix before heading off to see patients.

Breakfast Smoothie
8 ounces water (reverse-osmosis filtered)
½ cup frozen organic strawberries
1½ cup spinach
1 tablespoon of coconut oil
½ avocado

Blend for twenty to thirty seconds, and it will be ready to enjoy. This healthy smoothie will sustain you until lunchtime.

After drinking this, I will also have two cups of Bulletproof Coffee throughout the morning. See item 6 below for my Bulletproof Coffee recipe.

Lunches and Dinners

The theme for your lunches and dinners is largely green foods. Yes, green foods! If you want to live a long, healthy, and productive life, you absolutely have to focus your meals around greens and other vegetables. Vegetables contain a specific group of antioxidants called phytonutrients. I refer to them as plant nutrients, and I personally think of them as the fountain of youth.

There is no way around it; you have to eat your vegetables. So, keep your lunches and dinners simple, quick, and easy. You do not have to slave in the kitchen for an hour or two each night just to make dinner. If you love cooking that much, there is nothing wrong with taking your time in the kitchen. In fact, it may be therapeutic for you. But for most of us with families, jobs, and other obligations, that much time is just not available.

Here are some quick and easy dinner/lunch meals that you can start making tomorrow:

- Premade (bagged) salad topped with grilled chicken breast and a side of steamed asparagus.
- Naked burger topped with tomatoes, onions, and lettuce. Add a side of steamed broccoli or baked sweet potato fries.
- Veggie stir-fry: Throw all different sorts of chopped veggies into the skillet (using coconut oil).
  - PaleoHack 2.0 -Skip the soy sauce and use coconut aminos instead.
- Large Caesar salad: Add a bunch of cherry tomatoes, grapes, shredded carrots, and cabbage to have more substance, and make a bulkier meal than just a side salad.
- Spaghetti squash.

Kombucha Tea

Kombucha tea has been around for over a hundred years but has been noticed for its health properties over the past decade. What is kombucha tea? It is a functional drink made up of fermented green or black tea that can then be naturally sweetened with fruit and vegetable extracts. As we learned in chapter 6, consuming probiotics or healthy bacteria is essential for your entire body. Since kombucha is a fermented beverage, it contains healthy bacteria and yeast for your digestive tract that in turn will boost your immune-system function tremendously. I am a firm believer that most of us need to consume a probiotic supplement each and every day of our lives to reach maximum health, but eating and drinking fermented foods and drinks also can put you on the path to reaching your human potential.

My personal favorite brand is from a company called Synergy! It sells all different flavors of healthy kombucha tea such as strawberry, mango, and lemonade. Check them out; you can grab yours at your local grocery store or health-food store.

Fermented Foods (Vegetables)

Along the same lines as kombucha tea are fermented foods and vegetables. The most common fermented food that most Americans have heard of is sauerkraut, or fermented cabbage. Guess what? I hate the smell and the taste of it. If you disagree and actually like this stuff; start to eat it a lot. Use it as a side dish for dinner, or add it on top of salads and other healthy foods.

The good news is that there are a lot of other healthy fermented foods and vegetables on the market now. My favorite brand is Ozuke, which markets everything from fermented beets (YUM) to kimchi to citrus and ginger! As with kombucha tea, by consuming fermented foods and veggies, you are going to be feeding your intestines healthy bacteria that your body thrives on!

One of my favorite fermented treats is from a company called inner-eco. These are naturally effervescent, artisan crafted probiotic drinks made from coconut water with a delicious berry flavor. Each serving bursts with billions of active probiotic cultures. You can find these fermented, probiotic drinks at your local Whole Foods or other natural grocery stores throughout the country. For more info, check out their website at http://www.inner-eco.com.

Coconut

This is probably my favorite biohack. The power of coconuts is amazing. You have to start buying a coconut or two from your natural-foods store each week. Twice a week for breakfast, I share an entire coconut with my two daughters who are currently one and three years old and love coconuts even more than I do. After cutting open the coconut, we pour its water into glasses to drink. I have been referring to coconut water as nature's Gatorade for years. This stuff is superhydrating and loaded with electrolytes. It tastes great, and your kids will love it, too! After we get the coconut water out, I take a spoon and start to scrape out the coconut meat. The coconut meat tastes great and is very easily digested. The meat contains proteins, good fats, vitamins, and minerals. A coconut is the perfect storm for an extremely healthy breakfast. Besides eating and drinking the coconut, we use coconut oil every single day in our household; it is a staple in the *Non-Stop Paleo Life*.

Here's the deal with coconut oil: it is actually a solid at room temperature, so if you just want to consume it naturally like I do, you will have to get over the "texture thing." It's not a big deal, as it will melt right in your mouth. In the *Non-Stop Paleo Lifestyle*, I suggest you take a spoonful of coconut oil every day.

We have already talked about good fats, bad fats, good omega-3s, and bad omega-6s. Coconut oil contains a different kind of fat called medium-chain triglycerides or MCTs. These fats are extremely healthy for your brain, which uses them for fuel. By consuming coconut oil first thing in the morning, you are giving your brain the fuel it needs to be focused and efficient. This is something you will notice right away. Other benefits include the antibacterial, antifungal, and antiviral properties of coconut oil. When you feel a cold or flu coming on, take a couple spoonfuls of coconut oil throughout the day to help kill the bug.

Another great feature of coconut oil, unlike other oils, is you can actually heat it up and cook with it, and it will not become rancid. When you cook up other oils, the process can turn them into trans fats that are very detrimental to your health. I recommend that you cook with coconut oil exclusively. The only other oil I recommend consuming is olive oil, but—make no mistake about it—I would not heat it up. Use olive oil strictly for drizzling on salads and other steamed vegetables.

Here are some great uses for coconut oil:
Scrambled eggs
Omelets
Gluten-free and grain-free desserts
Veggies done in the skillet
Skin moisturizer
Antibacterial cream
An addition to popcorn on your cheat night
Coffee creamer
Topping on baked potatoes
Natural throat lozenges
Oil pulling for healthy mouth hygiene
Massage oil
Baby moisturizer for diaper rash

Bulletproof Coffee
I can cite many studies on the benefits of organic, black coffee. It is the most popular drink in the world. When taken in its natural form, coffee has many benefits, but now there is a much healthier and more effective way of drinking your morning cup of joe. At this point, I do

not think I have to even mention that you cannot be adding sugar, cream, syrups, chocolate, or artificial sweeteners to your morning coffee. I think we all understand that by now! Either drink it black or drink Bulletproof Coffee.

So exactly what is Bulletproof Coffee? Bulletproof Coffee was the creation of Dave Asprey, the founder and creator of the Bulletproof Diet and a fellow biohacker. Bulletproof Coffee will not only give you a morning or afternoon boost in energy, but it is extremely helpful to the brain's processing and focus. You will get more energy and feel less jittery by drinking Bulletproof Coffee rather than normal coffee or other caffeine products.

Here is how you make it. First, brew up a cup or two of organic coffee. I would also recommend that you use reverse-osmosis filtered water for your coffee (and all your drinking and cooking water). Next, put the coffee in your blender or Vitamix, and add a tablespoon of coconut oil and a tablespoon of unsalted, grass-fed butter. Blend for twenty to thirty seconds, and your new frothy and delicious morning health drink will be ready.

You will notice more energy, longer hours of focus, decreased appetite, and even therapeutic weight loss effects.

Non-Stop Paleohack 2.0: Don't have time or like the latte-like taste of Bulletproof Coffee? On my early workdays, before I go into the office, all I do is add a tablespoon of coconut oil to my cup of coffee and mix it in with a spoon. This only takes two seconds on the way out the door, but you still get the benefits of all the healthy fats in coconut oil right inside your morning cup of joe.

Bone Broth

Brain health, immune health, and longevity all start in your GUT. How do you get a healthy gut? You get a healthy gut by making bone broth every weekend and sipping on a cup of it every day. Bone broth is packed with minerals and nutrients to help stave off leaky-gut syndrome, help with your digestion, and give your stressed-out immune system a powerful boost. Start preparing bone broth each weekend, and sip on a cup every day.

Here is the link to my personal bone-broth recipe: http://www.nonstoppaleo.com/nonstoppaleo-recipes/bone-broth-recipe/.

Grass-Fed Meats

Simply put, if your meat is eating grains, then you are eating grains. You cannot be truly Paleo if you are getting any sort of grain in your diet, even if by indirect means. The best way to ensure that you're buying grass-fed meats is to buy in bulk from a local farm. This will help keep costs down, and you'll know exactly where your meat has come from. Get to know the farmer, form a good relationship, and let the farmer know exactly what you are looking for.

> *Meat has gotten a bad rap for a few decades. The problem isn't that meat is unhealthy for you. The problem lies within what the meat is eating. If your meat is eating grains, then you are eating grains.*
> *—Dr. Nick Caras*

It will be nice to go to the grocery store and skip the meat section every week, knowing that you have plenty of meat at home already.

Walking Every Day

During the Paleolithic time period, people walked all day every day. In today's world with computers and desk jobs, it's a little more difficult to get all your steps in. In the technological world we live in, though, there are many trackers, like Fitbits, that can track your steps. Get up and move on a daily basis. After dinner, don't go straight to the couch;

get outside and walk. Park in the back of the parking lot. Take the stairs instead of the elevator. Every little bit counts, and at end of the week, you will be better off for it.

Avocados on Everything

We should change the old saying "An apple a day keeps the doctor away" to "An avocado a day keeps the doctor away." These little treats are packed with nutrition. They are one of the best and easiest ways to get good fats into the diet and are also a great source of minerals and antioxidants. You can put them in smoothies, make guacamole, top your burger, or just eat them as a side dish with a little bit of sea salt and pepper. For babies, they are a great first solid food. Just mash them up into an applesauce consistency and give them to your infants.

Olive-Oil Drizzling (but no heating)

Olive oil is another great fat to keep in your diet on a regular basis. (So are olives.) The only problem with olive oil is that if it is heated, the fat becomes rancid. So only heat your coconut oil. But don't hesitate to drizzle olive oil on everything! From your morning omelets to salads and veggies, drizzle high-quality olive oil on different foods for taste, antioxidants, and healthy-fat content.

Non-Stop Paleohack 2.0: Do not buy olive oil in bulk. Every time you open the bottle, oxygen gets in and ruins the health benefits of olive oil. Buy the little bottles, and do not leave them open while you are cooking. Put the cap back on the bottle as soon as you are done using the olive oil.

Nuts and Seeds

Nuts and seeds are great healthy-fat sources for your everyday diet. They are a great biohack because they are Paleo, easy, and very satisfying, and the best part about it is they satisfy your daily "crunch" tooth (not be confused with sweet tooth!). I suggest grabbing a mixed bag of nuts and seeds because they all contain different amounts and types of nutrients and healthy fats. The only rule here is to stay away from peanuts as peanuts are detrimental to your health. All other nuts and seeds are OK. Keep a bag at work and, if you get hungry, grab a handful of nuts instead of some other processed or sugary snack. This little trick will keep your appetite satisfied throughout the day.

Non-Stop PaleoHack 2.0: Sneak a bag of nuts or healthy trail mix into the movie theater or your next sporting event so you will not be tempted to grab a bag of popcorn.

Cleaning the Entire House with Vinegar and Water

There are obviously a lot of toxins in the foods we eat, but some of the biggest sources of toxicity are lurking in your cleaning supplies. Whether it's your window cleaner, carpet cleaner, kitchen-counter cleaner, hardwood-floors cleaner, or even your personal cleaners, such as soaps and shampoos, there are hundreds of toxins in all of this stuff. You do not just eat toxins, you breathe them in, and they are absorbed through your skin as well. It's time to go green. Throw out all your current cleaning supplies, soaps, and lotions, and go all natural. The best cleaner for your home is to mix vinegar and water into an empty spray bottle. If you like scented cleaners, add in a couple drops of essential oils like lemon or orange. This will ensure you are reducing your toxic load and easing the toxin burden on your liver, kidneys, and entire body. Our Paleolithic ancestors never had the huge toxic burden that we do in the twenty-first century.

Walking Instead of Watching TV

Walking is so important that I included it twice in this chapter. I know we are all superbusy, and sometimes we just want to hit the couch after a long day of work. One of the best little paleohacks I can give you is to go walking after dinner. A thirty-minute walk each day helps prevent heart disease and cancer—America's biggest killers—by 60–80 percent. Just make this a habit: as soon as dinner is over, put on your walking shoes and take the family around the neighborhood. You will notice you will feel better, sleep better, and are more energized; it will even positively affect your mood. This is one of the easiest and most effective paleohacks you can start incorporating into your life right now.

Egg Yolk

Why do menus still have "egg-white omelets" on them? Egg yolk is a Paleo SuperFood that has gotten a bad rap over the past couple decades. From infants to adults, egg yolks do a body good. So quit skipping the yolk; it is actually more beneficial than the egg white. Make sure you are getting organic, free-range eggs to ensure the presence of a healthy dose of omega-3 fats, vitamins, and antioxidants. The perfect breakfast should contain protein and healthy fats; egg yolks will give you both.

Non-Stop Paleohack 2.0: Your baby's first food should be the egg yolk from a soft-boiled egg.

Cave Dwellers' Sense of Community

Make sure to do "this Paleo thing" together as a family. Your chances of success will be much higher. In our busy lives, we often push family and togetherness to the side because we are running around so much. Our "convenience" lifestyle has gotten in the way of our sense of community. Family, neighbors, friends, and even coworkers can all be a big part of your community and help you through life. Planning and carrying out the Paleo lifestyle in particular is much more enjoyable when doing it with loved ones, and research has shown that you will live longer and happier if you have a solid "community" around you.

*Make it more common to have friends
and family over for long dinners. It is
healthy for you and your soul.*
—Dr. Nick Caras

Getting Off Your Wi-Fi

Disconnect yourself from the world and escape the "emergency mode" that I feel we're in all day long. Every time your phone beeps, vibrates, or rings, you do not have to stop what you are doing and look at it. Make a list of your priorities and answer unexpected phone calls, e-mails, and texts later. Just as you schedule meetings, schedule a time to do those things. Most of them are meaningless anyway; rarely is a phone call an actual emergency. This will be one of the most liberating habits you can start today. Make yourself—not the outside world—the priority.

Getting in the Sun

Sunlight has gotten a bad rap as of late. Trust me, you need more of it. From hormones to skin health to vitamin-D levels to even your sleep, sunlight will help. Of course, you do not want to get out there and burn, but you do want a healthy tan. If you live in a place where there isn't much sun, think about investing in a healthy tanning bed. Your body will feel and look better, and your emotions will improve dramatically.

Resistance Training

It still kills me when people say they would rather do long-distance cardio training rather than some form of resistance training like weight-lifting. If you only have time to do one, opt for the weights. They will help you burn fat quicker and more efficiently and get you down to your ideal weight quicker than jogging around the track. Our Paleo ancestors were cross-fit trainers, and you should be too! Start hitting the weights and feel the burn; you'll notice the difference quickly.

Kale Chips

This is one of the easiest and healthiest paleohacks I can recommend. Simply take the kale off the stalk, throw the leaves onto a baking sheet and into the oven at 375 degrees for eight minutes, and sprinkle on some garlic salt; now you have a great snack. Everyone from toddlers to adults will love these little crunchy delights. Did I mention they are a powerhouse superfood loaded with antioxidants and nutrients? Enjoy!

Non-Stop Paleo Sleep

Sleep may be the most underrated or undertalked-about part of your overall health and well-being. Make better sleep a goal of yours over the next year. Here are a few hacks that will enhance your sleep tremendously. First of all, completely black out your room. Banish alarm clocks and Wi-Fi from the bedroom. Get blackout shades or curtains for your windows, because even the slightest light from underneath the door or from the moon can be problematic to your sleep cycle. Don't watch TV or use a computer or cell phone for at least an hour before bed. Read for around thirty minutes before bed in dim lighting. If you're still not sleeping properly, try an Epsom-salts bath before bed.

Non-Stop Paleohack 2.0: Get a healthy, nontoxic mattress. I personally recommend Intellibed to all my patients, which is made from nontoxic gel and not off-gassing foam.

Fats

Some believe that fat is a new fad, but it's not a fad at all. You see, we humans have been eating healthy fat for a long time. If something says

"Fat-Free" on it, just think chemical shit storm and run away as fast as you can! Now let me clarify: you need to be eating healthy fat, and you should be eating it every day and with every meal. Here are the best ones as far as I can tell:

- Olives
- Grass-fed meats
- Healthy fish
- Egg yolks
- Avocados
- Nuts (except peanuts)
- Grass-fed butter
- Seeds
- Coconuts
- Coconut oil
- Olive oil

Turmeric

Run out to your local health-food store right now, buy a bottle of this SuperFood seasoning and start sprinkling it on everything. This is the number-one researched herb, and its benefits are powerful. It is a heavy-duty, anti-inflammatory, antibacterial immune-system booster and cancer fighter, even though it will turn some of your food a little orange. You can marinade your meat in it before you put it on the grill, add it to smoothies, throw it on sautéed veggies, season your soups, and put it into almost any crockpot meal. It doesn't have much of a taste, but it is so powerful that my family tries to incorporate it into almost every dinner.

Start Each Meal with a Salad and/or Veggies

It's simple; we need vegetables, and we need a lot of them. They are packed with nutrients and vitamins and will help keep your body alkalized. It's hard to hear people complain that they don't get enough veggies because they have to eat out for work or they travel a lot for work. Every restaurant in the United States has a salad on the menu. You will be surprised at how many varieties and different types of salads you can have when you really start reading the menus. The more cut-up veggies in your salad, the better. Get different varieties to keep your body alkalized and healthy. At home, keep it simple by adding different proteins to your salads.

Non-Stop Paleohack 2.0: Opt for the side of veggies instead of the french fries, too.

Sprinting Instead of Jogging

Jogging is so 1980s. It is time to catch up with the latest and greatest research and start performing high-intensity cardio training. The days of putting on the running shoes and jogging around the block are over. It is unnecessary, time-consuming, and detrimental to your health. The research clearly shows that sprints are a much better way to exercise. Sprinting is better for your heart, lungs, entire cardiovascular system, immune system, and mental health, and the kicker is that it will help you shed pounds fast and effectively. So quit wasting hours per week on your morning jog; take a quick fifteen minutes to do some sprints, and you will be better off for it. This paleohack will save you a few hours per week.

Smoothies

If you do smoothies right, they can be a power-packed breakfast or meal replacement. No more excuses that you do not have enough time in the morning for a nutritious breakfast: there are plenty of healthy and delicious recipes out there. Unfortunately, a lot of people make "sugar bombs" out of their smoothies. The biggest mistake you can make with regard to smoothies is using some sort of juice for its base. Here is a quick sample smoothie: start with some water; add in a couple handfuls of spinach or kale; and throw in a couple cups of frozen berries, a scoop of coconut oil, a healthy protein powder, and fiber powder, and maybe add in fruit and vegetable powder as well (as I like to do). If you like your smoothies thick, try also putting in an avocado or coconut yogurt.

> *There is nothing easier you can start doing for yourself right now than making a daily smoothie.*
> *—Dr. Nick Caras*

Goals, Affirmations, and Journaling

I call this one "Paleo thinking." I believe we are under so much stress in this day and age from job stress, home stress, financial worries, and keeping up with the Joneses that we need to calm down our brains, minds, and nervous systems on a daily basis. I believe one of the best ways to do this is to start the morning off right by doing some sort of positive mental visualization. This can take the form of writing down your goals, saying affirmations, or journaling. Others prefer to meditate or pray. Find what works for you and stick with it. The main theme here is to do it every single morning. There are many benefits of these types of activities, and they will definitely get your day started off on the right foot. If you stay consistent with this practice, you will be amazed by how much success, happiness, and joy come into your life.

Non-Stop Paleohack 2.0: Bedtime journaling. A great way to help you sleep better and release stress before bedtime is journaling right before you go to bed. Put all your thoughts and tomorrow's goals down on paper. This will help ease your mind for a better night's sleep.

Drinking Nothing but Water

Guess what? If you want to lose weight and lose it fast, try this little hack. For thirty days straight, do not change anything in your normal food intake or exercise routine, but don't drink anything other than water—and watch the magic happen. This means no coffee, no juice, and no alcohol: nothing but Water! By just changing your liquid intake, you will lose weight, clear your skin, and flush out toxic junk from your liver, kidneys, and colon. Magic will happen once you start drinking nothing else but good ol' H_2O. This is an easy one: I suggest you give it a try and start today.

Eating Prior to Work Functions and Other Parties

One of the biggest excuses I hear from my patients and clients is that they are too busy to stay Paleo or they simply have too much going on. They have work outings, family get-togethers, and other social events. There are always food and drinks being thrown at them at all these events and gatherings. The fact of the matter is that it takes a little willpower and planning to stay Paleo in our hectic lives. A quick little hack is to eat at home before you go out to all your different functions. This will give you a little more willpower to say no to the appetizer plate.

Non-Stop Paleohack 2.0: If you know you have a work function or social gathering on, say, Thursday night, use your one cheat meal of the week for that. Weekly planning and goal-setting is essential to keep yourself on track.

Lemon or Lime in Your Water

Super easy hack! Every time you go to the grocery store, make sure to grab some organic limes and/or lemons. At home, slice them up and throw a slice in each glass of water you consume. Along with the great taste, the citrus is alkalizing to your system, which will help with every-thing from digestion to energy levels to immune health! It's simple, easy, and effective—no excuses for not trying this easy paleohack!

Saying NO to Alcohol

I like to have fun as much as the next person, but we should all take a break from alcohol every so often. My challenge to you is to take a month off from alcohol. If you're just starting Paleo, you should take off at least one month. Alcohol is acidic, causes leaky gut, and just warps your energy levels. It is also a big burden on your liver and kid-neys. It's time to take a break. You can read some more info at www. NonStopPaleo.com on how to do alcohol the right way; but why not challenge yourself and take a thirty-day break? It will be good for your body, mind, and soul.

Non-Stop Paleo Pasta

Translation: **Spaghettis squash or zucchini pasta with hearty, meaty sauces.** We all like a good bowl of pasta every so often. Here is a good way to do a guilt-free pasta night. Find out which sort of noodles you personally like better between spaghetti-squash or zucchini pasta, and then make the sauce a complete, health-enhancing Superfood. Grab some organic, grass-fed beef or buffalo, your favorite veggies, herbs and tomato sauce, and dig in. It will feel like cheat-meal comfort food but offer all the benefits of a Paleo Super Meal!

Sprouting

Sprouting is one of the easiest, most affordable, and best ways to eat your vegetables. In fact, sprouts can have up to thirty times the num-ber of nutrients than the vegetable itself. Anyone can grow sprouts anywhere. We actually grow sprouts in our own kitchen every week.

You can put sprouts on almost any dish to add more phytonutrients to your meals. You can throw them into your smoothies, scrambled eggs, omelets, salads, and soups, or even garnish marinades for meat and fish.

Crockpots

Crockpotting meals is one of the essentials in our household. In our busy lifestyle involving work and kids, we find there is no easier way to prepare an extremely healthy meal with plenty of SuperFoods than by using a crockpot. From healthful chilies, soups, and other protein-based meals, to bone broths, you can put your ingredients in your crockpot at noon and find that dinner will be ready at 5:00 p.m., with no dinnertime prep work necessary. This is one of the ways you can stay on track during a busy work week.

Nontoxic Mattresses

Your mattress is one of the most toxic pieces of furniture in your entire house. Most mattresses are made from foam, a substance that off-gasses. You actually breathe in toxic fumes while you are sleeping. Ever wonder why you cannot get a good night's sleep? This may be the reason. I highly suggest you switch to a nonfoam mattress immediately. You will sleep better because you will breathe better all night long. I personally recommend either a cotton mattress or a gel mattress.

Non-Stop Paleohack 2.0: I recommend Intellibed mattresses, which my entire family sleeps on. If you would like to order one, go to www.intellibed.com and enter the code **DrCaras** to receive 10 percent off your new mattress.

Intermittent Fasting

Over the years, one of my main goals has been to find information on what can help you live longer while feeling great. Research has shown that fasting can actually turn on your longevity DNA. Intermittent fasting is actually much easier than you think. How it works is that you only eat during a six- to eight-hour span throughout the day. For example, you may consume your meals from around 11:00 a.m. to 6:00 p.m. So basically, you have a decent lunch, a healthy afternoon snack, and a healthy dinner, and then you will not eat again until lunch the next day. Drink as much water throughout the day as you wish; after a couple days your morning hunger pangs will go away and you will start to feel reenergized and much healthier. You do not have to do this all the time, but a couple days a week or maybe every other week will help out your health levels tremendously.

CHAPTER 10

Non-Stop: Putting It All Together

I would personally like to congratulate you on making it to the end of *The Non-Stop Paleo Life*. You have taken a huge step in your health and longevity. You now have the tools to help you age gracefully and enjoy a long life with extreme health, happiness, energy, production, and abundance. Start putting the tools you have learned to work immediately. The quicker you can get from point A to point B, the more likely you will want to stick with the *Non-Stop Paleo Life* program. Have fun trying out new recipes, new exercises, and new ways of thinking. Get your essential blood work taken and get a baseline. Chapter 6 shows you exactly what tests you should ask your doctor to order. After three to six months, get yourself retested to see how much progress you have made. Go to your local functional-medicine doctor or my online vitamin and supplement store at http://drnick.metagenics.com/store and pick up the supplements I have laid out in chapter 6 as well. Start them immediately to reap their benefits.

The exercises and the diet part of the *Non-Stop Paleo* program are self-explanatory. People miss the boat on lifestyle changes because they do not attempt to change their thought processes. Revisit the section on "Non-Stop Paleo Thinking" in chapter 4, and start a routine to change the way you think. If your mind and attitude aren't on board, it is going to be hard to stick with a lifestyle change. Habits are embedded in all of us at a very young age. Whether they came from our parents, our teachers, or our coaches, they become engrained in our nervous systems. Changing bad habits and undoing bad lifestyle choices will be a continual battle. Of course, we can all change for a week or a month, but what I really want for you is a positive change for the rest of your life. A lot of research states that it takes ninety days to turn a specific change into a lifestyle. You do not have to perform all the suggestions about Paleo thinking habits, but find out which ones resonate with you and make a daily practice of them.

> *Patients are always looking for a magic bullet, a new pill, or a new lotion that will give them more energy and better health. There isn't a magic bullet you can buy. You have to EARN health and energy. You have to earn your health.*
> *—Dr. Nick Caras*

The lifestyle blueprint offered here is something that will not change. Even as technology advances and we find out more about the human body and how all the cells in our bodies work, I am confident that the suggestions in this book will not change. Our DNA doesn't really change. Healthy habits will always feed our DNA and help us live longer. Sure, we may find out about other healthy habits that our Paleolithic ancestors practiced, and we can incorporate those habits, but what we know now is a great guide to being as healthy as possible. Keep this book close to you and revisit it as you progress through your new lifestyle. Like all of us, you will always be able to be a little better. The habits and lifestyle changes in this book will get easier as you progress.

All the paleohacking tips in chapter 9 are there to make your life easier. We all live very busy and hectic lives. There is never enough time in the day to get everything done. Often we take time and life for granted. Occasionally, we should step back and see how precious life really is. As a father of two with a full-time job, I know how stressful it may be to try to do things right all of the time. Paleohacking tricks will help put time back in your day and keep your physiology healthy. There is a happy medium out there that allows you to be productive and healthy at the same time. Plus, we have built-in cheat days and cheat meals as well. This is the major premise of *Non-Stop Paleo*: it has to be nonstop for the rest of your life, not just for next month. Start to live by the 90/10 rule we talked about in chapter 1. Remember your goals and your motivations. Why do you want to be healthy? Why do you want to live a long life? Why do you want to have more energy? Why do you want to lose weight? Only you can answer these questions. You must know your why or you will neither make a lifestyle change nor continue to live by the 90/10 rule. Enjoy your cheat meals; you deserve them. Don't feel guilty about them. Life is never long enough; it is OK to enjoy the time we have.

One Last Piece of Advice

Make this a family affair. It is never too early to teach your children about living a healthful lifestyle. Follow the *Non-Stop Paleo* guidelines with your entire family. The first few years of life are vitally important to the development of children's immune systems. You have the ability to set them up for success and health for the rest of their lives. I believe that as a parent, it is our obligation to get our kids off to a healthy start. If you do not have a family, get healthy with your spouse. If you are single, share the program with a friend and do it together. Hold yourself and each other accountable, and you will get better results. It is always much more fun to get healthy with someone else.

It is my sincere hope that you have learned something from this book and that you are willing to put that something into action. Start today! Every choice you make is either putting you closer to health or closer to disease. Start making the healthier choices! If you need more help and more guidance, check out: http://www.nonstoppaleo.com/paleo-lifestyle-8-week-bootcamp/.

The 8 week BootCamp will guide you through weekly, in-depth videos about how to implement the strategies laid out in this book. If you feel you are self-motivated and can start implementing the Non-Stop Paleo Life today, just go ahead and get started. But if you need a little more guidance, check out the website. Remember, the most important thing is that you just get started.

I wish you luck in your journey to health. Remember that you only have one life to live and that life is the most beautiful thing in the world. Take advantage of it, embrace it, enjoy it, and make it the best life possible through Non-Stop Paleo. Very good things will soon follow. The only reason that I know what I know today about health, wellness, and longevity is that I refused to quit learning. I continue to refuse to take Western medicine as the only answer. I urge you to keep reading and learning about the Paleo lifestyle. When you are not sure about something, just ask yourself if you think your ancestors would have done this, or eaten that. Even the guidance in this book is not the only answer—and yours is not the only question—but it gives you a good start. I believe the Paleo lifestyle is the best way to live, and I am enjoying every second of my life. Jump on board, and you will love your results as well.

Again, good luck with your new journey as you start the rest of your life today.
Yours in True Health and Wellness,
Dr. Nick Caras

DR. CARAS'S ADVANCED PROGRAMS

Leaky-Gut Program

If you are trying to get rid of your leaky gut, Dr. Caras's revolutionary program will provide some of the most important information you'll ever read. With many years of clinical practice under his belt and having treated thousands of patients with leaky-gut syndrome, Dr. Caras finally decided to put this program down on paper for you.

Dr. Caras has a simple goal of helping as many people as possible get rid of leaky gut and keep it away for the rest of their lives. His goal does come with one caveat, though. He doesn't want you to cover up your leaky gut through medications or a hoax diet plan; he wants you to get rid of your leaky gut for good—by all-natural remedies. You see, it's actually fairly simple once you know how to eliminate, fertilize, and reinoculate with very specific, all-natural strategies that Dr. Caras has been testing repeatedly with much success.

We are not promising a quick fix in just a couple days or even a week, as many bogus sites do. We all know that fad diets and a "secret super vitamin" do not exist. If they did, we all would be signing up. Dr. Caras's program is four weeks long and contains very specific and exact strategies to follow.

Just imagine a healthier gut in just thirty days. Just imagine weight falling off, better digestion, a more optimally working immune system, and no more allergies and sinus issues. However your symptoms are showing up, isn't it time to get rid of them once and for all?

What You Will Learn

- How to fertilize your gut
- What specific prebiotics and probiotics you need to take
- What you need to start eating and drinking today
- Which select group of foods causes leaky gut

- The number-one superfood that gets rid of leaky-gut syndrome
- Dr. Caras's number-one leaky-gut superfood recipe
- How to increase the growth of your "good" bacteria
- How to "moisturize" your gut lining
- And much, much more

To gain access to Dr. Caras's leaky-gut program, go to:

http://www.nonstoppaleo.com/get-rid-of-leaky-gut/.

PALEO LIFESTYLE EIGHT-WEEK BOOTCAMP

Learn how to feel and look your best in just eight weeks. Dr. Caras has helped thousands of people in private practice since 2004. His book *Detoxify Your Lifestyle* has helped even more people live a healthy life in the United States and around the globe. Now, Dr. Caras's PALEO Lifestyle BootCamp has put together everything you need to take your health back in just eight weeks.

Dr. Caras will break it down for you in weekly videos. Each week, he will add in a new healthy Paleo protocol for you to implement in your life and your family's life. Yours will be the healthiest family on your block with the BootCamp.

This Is Why I Put Together the Paleo Lifestyle Eight-Week BootCamp

When I realized you needed a little more than just a book or a seminar, I worked day and night to put together this program. We live in a sick and toxic world. The United States is one of the unhealthiest industrialized countries in the world. We take more medications than any other country in the world, yet we still rank as one of the unhealthiest (go figure). Only YOU are responsible for your own health. It is time that YOU take responsibility and start getting healthy TODAY.

This Program Is for You, if You:

- Are sick and tired of being sick and tired
- Want to follow an entire PALEO Lifestyle (not just the diet)
- Are chronically ill and ready for a change
- Have tried everything and still feel like crap
- Are ready for a new lease on life for yourselves and your families

- Want more happiness
- Want more energy
- Want a better relationship with food and with yourself
- Want to be able to fall asleep and stay asleep for an entire night
- Need more passion and purpose in your life

This Program Is NOT for You, if You:

- Have a quick-fix mentality
- Have a fad-diet mentality
- Are lazy
- Want to rely on your doctor for a new magic pill, potion, or lotion
- Like to blame your doctor for all your ailments
- Want to blame genetics (DNA) instead of overcoming them
- Are not willing to change your lifestyle habits

For more information or to purchase the program, follow the link below:

http://www.nonstoppaleo.com/paleo-lifestyle-8-week-bootcamp/.

HEALTH, WELLNESS, AND PEAK-PERFORMANCE CONSULTATION WITH DR. CARAS

Do you still have health concerns and questions that need to be answered? Do you want to know the right foods to consume for your specific condition? Are you wondering what specific vitamins and nutrients you need? Would you like to know the keys to peak athletic performance? Have you ever wondered why you cannot lose the weight even though you are eating right and exercising? Do you have other health questions that haven't been answered?

Here is your chance to talk to a real health practitioner, Dr. Caras, on a one-hour phone consultation. Any and all your questions will be answered. The floor is yours for approximately one hour. We can go through any health and wellness question or topic of your concern. Your health history, your exercise routines, your diet plan, your stress, your family history, and so forth. No stone will be left unturned.

Dr. Caras has helped thousands of patients lose weight, find a balanced life, relieve stress, and reach their peak potential. You owe it to yourself to learn how to break through whatever is holding you back. Whether you're concerned with your blood work, X-rays, MRIs, or other indicators, Dr. Caras will thoroughly go through all your previous tests with you and guide you on your way to health and wellness.

Dr. Caras charges thousands of dollars in private practice to treat his patients but is currently scheduling his one-hour phone consultations for only $199.

Check out the link below for more information:

http://www.nonstoppaleo.com/health-wellness-peak-performance-consultation-with-dr-caras/.

SEVEN-DAY KETOGENIC DIET PLAN

Why should you try the SEVEN-DAY KETOGENIC DIET PLAN?

To sum it all up, this diet plan will put your body into extreme fat-burning mode. Do you need to LOSE WEIGHT fast? There is no better way than getting your body into a "state of ketosis."

What is ketosis?

Simply put, when you take all the carbohydrates out of your body, your body has nothing else to burn up besides fat. When this happens, you have entered a state of ketosis. This is when you go into FAT-BURNING OVERDRIVE!

Not only will you start to **lose weight fast**; you will also:

- Have increased energy
- Lose your cravings
- Boost your immune system
- Improve thyroid health
- Sleep better
- Digest your food better
- Improve your brain health

and so much more. If you are ready to finally try out the ketogenic diet, I have put together a simple seven-day plan just for you.

The ketogenic diet isn't something you have to do all the time, but periodically getting your body into ketosis throughout the year will help it in so many ways. Most importantly, it will keep your body's metabolism in check so you can look your best and keep the nasty pounds off as you age.

For just $11.99, you can download Dr. Caras's ketogenic-diet plan right now! Go to this link for the instant download:

http://www.nonstoppaleo.com/ketogenic-diet-plan/

SEVEN-DAY DETOX DIET PLAN

- Are you feeling sluggish?
- Do you need to kick-start your diet?
- Do you feel like you are on toxic overload?
- Do you have trouble sleeping; are you feeling fatigued?
- Do you feel bloated all the time?
- Are you just in a rut mentally, physically, and emotionally?

If you answered yes to any of these questions, it is time you take a week for yourself to DETOX. Detoxification is a very powerful way to reboot your body's systems so everything can work more efficiently.

Living in this day and age, we are constantly bombarded with toxins that put a HUGE burden on our liver, kidneys, thyroid, intestines, and many other organs and systems of the body. This toxic burden causes our body to weaken, making us more susceptible to weight gain, sickness, and disease.

Detoxing is a quick and easy way to lose weight, reset your metabolism, and get out of your rut. I have been teaching detox protocols and cleanses for over fifteen years in my private practice, and I have finally put together my best seven-day detox program just for people like you.

If you can commit seven days, then you can detox and begin feeling renewed and rejuvenated by next week.

Commit to your health and well-being by grabbing my latest and greatest seven-day detox blueprint, and take another step on your journey to looking and feeling your best!

For only $17.99, you can start detoxing today! Go to the link below for the instant download:

http://www.nonstoppaleo.com/7-day-detox-diet-plan/.

AUTHOR BIOGRAPHY

Dr. Nick Caras is an author, chiropractor, and health coach who has helped thousands of individuals from all over the world regain complete control of their health. Dr. Caras currently resides and practices in Highlands Ranch, Colorado, with his wife and two beautiful daughters. The Non-Stop Paleo Life is a follow-up to Dr. Caras's 2008 best-selling book Detoxify Your Lifestyle. Dr. Caras's mission is simple: to teach people what true health is and where it comes from. Our ancestors from the Paleolithic Era left clues, and Dr. Caras has put those clues together in one lifestyle plan and named the plan accordingly. If you are wondering how to incorporate the Paleo lifestyle in the busy, technological age that we live in, The Non-Stop Paleo Life is the blueprint for you.

For more information, visit www.NonStopPaleo.com.

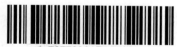